PRAISE FOR *VERY GENEROUS THINGS, PLANTS—WE DON'T DESERVE THEM, REALLY*

"This compilation of Christopher Hedley's stories, anecdotes and comments delightfully conveys his unique wisdom on herbs and the people that need them. You will find it an easy read, with a quirky humour that will make you laugh out loud. But make no mistake, its simplicity conveys profound understanding. Christopher was surely the most influential UK herbalist of his time, and this book will enable future herbalists to benefit from his wisdom as we did."

Robyn Soma, President of the National Institute of Medical Herbalists

"This book is not only an academic text but is an engaging and thought-provoking insight into the philosophy and practice of Christopher Hedley, master herbalist. It is an autobiography enriched with the stories and anecdotes of his lifelong devotion to plants and people within his practice. As a notable scholar of humoral medicine and traditional herbal practice his doctrine is based on an understanding of the unique physiology and lifestyle of the person and the importance of matching the herb to the patient."

Dr Julie Whitehouse, Principal Lecturer of Herbal Medicine, University of Westminster (retired)

"There is no way of describing the actual truth of things, so we have to approach it sideways with stories. If you resonate with these words from Christopher, you will love this book. Playful, insightful, informative and highly readable, it is a peach of a book. It is filled with unique and personal pointers on the road to herbal practice, is brimming with memorable ways to befriend plants, and radiates love for people and plants, just like its author. Christopher inspired generations of herbalists, and this book will continue that process."

Keith Robertson MSc. FNIMH, Director of Education, Scottish School of Herbal Medicine

VERY GENEROUS THINGS, PLANTS— WE DON'T DESERVE THEM, REALLY

VERY GENEROUS THINGS, PLANTS—WE DON'T DESERVE THEM, REALLY

Stories, Anecdotes and Nuggets of Wisdom from Herbalist Christopher Hedley

Edited by
Guy Waddell
with a foreword by bendle

AEON

First published in 2025 by
Aeon Books

Copyright © 2025 by Christopher Hedley

The right of Christopher Hedley to be identified as the author of this work has been asserted in accordance with §§ 77 and 78 of the Copyright Design and Patents Act 1988.

All rights reserved. No part of this publication may be reproduced, stored in a retrieval system, or transmitted, in any form or by any means, electronic, mechanical, photocopying, recording, or otherwise, without the prior written permission of the publisher.

British Library Cataloguing in Publication Data

A C.I.P. for this book is available from the British Library

ISBN-13: 978-1-80152-184-0

Typeset by Medlar Publishing Solutions Pvt Ltd, India

www.aeonbooks.co.uk

CONTENTS

FOREWORD by bendle	xiii
INTRODUCTION by Guy Waddell	xvii
Roots—Resourcing Humoral Thinking for Plant Medicine	3
The Choleric Humour	3
They'll get up and walk out	3
It just came out	4
It's tough	5
Move your body	5
Do you want a recipe?	5
Introduce the idea	6
Just pretend	6
Scattered fire	7
Really strong and solid in the centre	7
Two tissues	8
Jump off mountains	8
But then it's over	8

The Sanguine Humour	8
Extra bouncy	8
New things	9
Talking airy people into getting better	9
Air settles eventually	9
Just like that	9
Catapults in the front room	10
Sanguinosity	10
The only person to cycle up that hill	11
Began to eat	12
Turmeric hair	13
The Phlegmatic Humour	13
Fluxions of rheum	13
Cheese and pepper	14
Damn, I've had my leg shot off	14
Beware of angry phlegmatics	15
Water sinks	15
Two big things	15
Phlegmatocity	16
Be friendly and move on	16
It's a job to remember	17
Hydraulic engines	17
The Melancholy Humour	18
Melilot haze	18
Out to the heavens	18
What do you expect, really	18
Permission granted	19
You can upset an earthy person	19
Unsticking an astrologer	19
Like rocks	20
New ways	20
Let's face it	21
Walk four hundred miles	21
Dual-function thistles for Eeyore	21
The Humours Together	22
Is	22
Express yourself	22
Shape shifting	22
Comfort and calm	23

Being run over by a truck	23
A United Nations decree	24
Flowers—Materia Medica of Plant Medicine	**27**
Artist's Bracket (*Ganoderma applanatum*)	27
Must be soupy	27
Host to host	28
Astragalus (*Astragalus mongholicus* syn. *A. membranaceus*)	29
Approaching sideways with a story	29
Balm, Lemon Balm (*Melissa officinalis*)	29
We didn't have nerves	29
Bittersweet (*Solanum dulcamara*)	30
Six inches	30
Boneset (*Eupatorium perfoliatum*)	30
Poured it down his throat	30
Borage (*Borago officinalis*)	31
How happy they are	31
Cayenne (*Capsicum annuum* syn. *C. frutescens*)	32
He was red	32
Chaste Berry (*Vitex agnus-castus*)	32
Monk's pepper grinder	32
A funny feeling	32
Herbs change lives	33
Comfrey (*Symphytum officinale*)	33
People and cats	33
Nibbling up	34
Cramp Bark (*Viburnum opulus*)	35
Go by the smell	35
Echinacea, Coneflower (*Echinacea* spp.)	35
Even on herbalists themselves	35
Pushy regimes	36
Need a good vitality to work with	36
Disordered or loose heat	37
Elecampane (*Inula helenium*)	37
Chunky	37
A big hacking cough	38
All lung diseases	38
Elfshot	39
It's quite horrible	40

Ephedra (*Ephedra sinica*) — 40
    Take ten students — 40
Fennel (*Foeniculum vulgare*) — 41
    It tells us quite a lot — 41
Figwort (*Scrophularia nodosa* and *S. aquatica*) — 41
    The King's evil and a great hope for Charles — 41
Fly Agaric (*Amanita muscaria*) — 42
    A loss of scale — 42
    We could expect no less — 43
    True of all herbs — 44
Garlic (*Allium sativum*) — 44
    The simplest solution — 44
    A little pipe — 45
    Garlic addresses that — 45
    Appropriates to the human — 45
Ginkgo (*Ginkgo biloba*) — 46
    How Ginkgo leaves got their shape — 46
    Balances the immediate effect — 47
    Clottiness — 47
Goat's Rue (*Galega officinalis*) — 48
    Feeling better — 48
Golden Seal (*Hydrastis canadensis*), Barberry (*Berberis vulgaris*), Mahonia (*Berberis aquifolium*) — 49
    I try my best — 49
Greater Celandine (*Chelidonium majus*) — 50
    If you give enough of it — 50
Hawthorn (*Crataegus* spp.) — 50
    Takes longer, of course — 50
    Addressing fear — 51
    Start low — 52
    Agree in no time at all — 52
    The issue is redness — 53
    Clearing remedy — 53
    Like a good bouncer — 54
    That pleased me — 54
Herb Bennet, Wood Avens (*Geum urbanum*) — 55
    Rampant in my garden — 55
    Slightly different direction — 55
Hops (*Humulus lupulus*) — 56
    Hop babies — 56

Horsetail (*Equisetum arvense*) ... 56
    The minerals contribute ... 56
    I am happy with the tincture ... 57
Juniper (*Juniperus communis*) ... 57
    Black furry shapes ... 57
Kelp (including *Fucus vesiculosus*) ... 58
    Tip people over ... 58
Lady's Mantle (*Alchemilla vulgaris, A. mollis*) ... 58
    The lady in the sweet shop ... 58
    I use that term with affection and respect ... 59
    Mainstay ... 60
    It worked really well ... 60
    Not actually dew ... 61
Lily of the Valley (*Convallaria majalis*) ... 61
    Disturbance of the Shen too ... 61
    Subtle aspects of bitterness ... 62
    It doesn't hold like Hawthorn does ... 62
    Just a little tool ... 63
    Keep the heart ticking over ... 63
Lime Flowers (*Tilia* spp.) ... 64
    Four limes ... 64
Mayweed (*Anthemis cotula*) ... 64
    A lovely piece of disused railway line ... 64
Milk Thistle (*Silybum marianum* syn. *Carduus marianus*) ... 65
    Operation put off ... 65
    Runs under me when I sit down ... 65
Motherwort (*Leonurus cardiaca*) ... 66
    Within about ten seconds ... 66
Mugwort (*Artemisia vulgaris*) ... 67
    Save on the cinema sort of dreaming ... 67
    That's what Mugwort does ... 68
    My advertising sign ... 68
Myrhh (*Commiphora molmol*) ... 69
    I had a dream ... 69
Nettle (*Urtica dioica*) ... 70
    Phlegmatic superfluities ... 70
    In love with them ... 71
    Only a veneer ... 71
    All-time favourite ... 71

Passion Flower (*Passiflora incarnata*) 72
    Simple joys 72
Pellitory of the Wall (*Parietaria judaica*) 72
    Rearranging itself 72
Peony (*Paeonia lactiflora*) 73
    Being a serious herbalist 73
Peppermint (*Mentha x piperita*) 73
    Four actions 73
Plantain (*Plantago major, P. lanceolata*) 74
    I'll try and track this down 74
    The verticality of Plantains 74
    Bloody brilliant 75
Polypody of the Oak (*Polypodium vulgare*) 75
    It sinks down 75
Prickly Ash (*Zanthoxylum americanum, Z. clava-herculis*) 75
    Must be your circulation 75
Raspberry Leaf (*Rubus ideaus*) 76
    A soft furry blanket 76
    A bit grumbly in the tummy 77
Rhubarb (*Rheum officinale, R. palmatum*) 78
    A nice young man as well 78
Rose (*Rosa* spp.) 78
    You could liberate them 78
Rosebay Willowherb, Fireweed (*Epilobium angustifolium*) 79
    Left to itself, it heals 79
Rosemary (*Salvia rosmarinus* syn. *Rosmarinus officinalis*) 79
    From the heart outwards 79
    The Queen of Hungary and the Prince of Poland 80
    Continuities 81
Sage (*Salvia officinalis*) 81
    Holds energy in the centre 81
    Nice combination 82
    Empty heat 82
    Just think about the patient 83
    Sage helps deal with that 83
    By degrees 83
    Chew 84
    Sage total capacity point 84
    Leaf between leaves 85
    A reasonable strategy 85

And she did	85
Really strong, good smelling Sage	86
I'll let you know	86
St John's Wort (*Hypericum perforatum*)	87
With consistently good results	87
Feet firmly on the ground	87
Omelettes and amulets	88
You turn round and it disappears	88
A wort for St John	88
Skullcap (*Scutellaria lateriflora, S. galericulata*)	89
Single most useful herb in psychosis	89
Valerian (*Valeriana officinalis*)	89
A nineteenth century French cavalry officer	89
It will revolt	89
Vervain (*Verbena officinalis*)	90
The noise level goes up	90
Letting go	90
Might not finish the cup	91
Wormwood (*Artemisia absinthium*)	91
Charming, not	91
Seeds—Living Plants and Philosophy of Practice for Plant Medicine	93
My favourite bit	93
It's wonderful	93
It's a good exercise	94
Spending time	94
You can actually make it up	95
Three inches off the ground	95
Always	95
Totally possible	95
Donuts	95
Tradition and direct knowing	96
Feel better	97
Three names	97
Why do you ask?	97
You're my best friend	98
Canadian Fleabane on a busy road	98
Choosing herbs	99
When with patients	99

The third floor of the Natural History Museum	99
A very good understanding of biochemistry	100
Make a tea	100
Pushed down	100
Anybody could have done it	101
The plants themselves	102
It won't let me use it	102
The way she uses the herb	102
Even you and me	103
Slingbacks or open-toed sandals	104
Make it up as you go along	104
Two rules in herbal medicine	104
Become a different person	105
All that matters	105
Shut both eyes	106
Your own	106
Best medicine	106
You just describe it	107
I want to be a Victorian vicar	107
Egg-sucking	108
Studying the herb itself	108
In search of a trunk	108
Up until that point	109
Storing sunsets	109
How the plant is in the world	110
How it be	110
Adopting ancestors	111
Ineffable mystery	111
More baggy here	111
I shouldn't worry	112
Most together	112
One degree under	112
Get below	113
Really	114
REFERENCES	115
INDEX	119

FOREWORD

by bendle

I first met Non and Chris in the early 1980s when I was one of three people attending their first introductory class in herbal medicine. Later, Chris would teach similar classes for several years at the Mary Ward Centre in Central London, but this trial run was in the front room of their house. Chris did most of the teaching, although Non offered wise interjections and also fed us with homemade soup. I had previously given up attending a badly taught evening class in the same subject, but I loved these sessions. They gave me a framework for understanding the herbal lore I had been learning from books and inspired me to study more about the subject.

We got on well and I stayed in touch. At the time I was very involved with the London Musician's Collective based in a building just along the road from Non and Chris's place so I would often pop in for a chat when I was there. A few years later, when I was studying to be a herbalist myself, I sat in on some of Chris's consultations with patients in their home.

Non and Chris studied herbal medicine together, but Chris was the one who had originally enrolled on the training course and whose name was on the qualification. Chris defined his work as being a herbalist, whilst Non's practice was more eclectic, incorporating art therapy and massage. Unwilling to be pinned down with a label, she used to say, "a Non does what a Non does". While Chris gradually became more and more visible in the world as a teacher of herbal medicine, his teaching was very much rooted in his discussions with Non at home. Together they were herbalists 24 hours a day—sometimes literally, with Chris keeping daytime hours and Non studying and working through the night.

They lived and worked in a small basement flat in North London, near Chalk Farm. To enter their flat, one had to descend a metal stairway from the street to their front door. Inside the door there was a corridor which sometimes served as a waiting room—there was a chair for patients and a bookshelf. The first door in the corridor opened to a small room with a toilet and the second door opened onto their consulting room, which was also their dispensary. In this room, Chris or Non would sit on a chair with their patient seated on a settee. At the far end of the corridor was another door into the private part of their flat. There was a crowded small front room with an offshoot kitchen and stairs leading up to the ground floor part of their dwelling. French windows from the front room opened onto a small garden bordered by three high walls. Beyond the high wall facing the house ran the main railway line heading North from Euston station.

I had been visiting the flat for some years before I asked how many rooms were upstairs. I learned that there was only a bathroom up there. "But where do you sleep?", I asked. It was only at that point that I realised that their consultation room was also their bedroom. The settee upon which their patients sat was at the end of the day folded out into a double bed. So, as I mentioned, they were 24-hour herbalists, sleeping and dreaming with the echoes and energies of their patients' presence.

In the tiny yard at the front of their property they grew a huge cactus-like euphorbia reaching up to street level. In their backyard they grew a number of plants, but the space was very small. Despite living in urban North London for the 35 years that I knew him, Chris had an amazing knowledge of wild plants and fungi. He lived close to Regents Park and Primrose Hill and, slightly further afield, Hampstead Heath, where he would find and sometimes pick plants. He also loved finding things growing on neglected bits of "wasteland", in churchyards, carparks and emerging out of the towpath of the nearby Grand Union Canal.

Chris seemed, sometimes, to conjure plants into existence, and he instantly recognised unusual species. I remember one springtime, at a "munumunuh[1]" conference in Cirencester, he asked me if I had noticed

---

[1] Munumunuh = MNIMH—Member of the National Institute of Medical Herbalists

the vernal figwort growing near a path. I knew several species of figwort but had never previously heard of this one. At the same conference he shared with a group of us the knowledge about the jumping anthers in species of Berberis plants mentioned later in this book. I emulated his habit of always missing one session at herbal conferences to wander off and meet the local plants.

Sometimes Chris would take his patients out for a walk, pointing out living specimens of plants that were in their medicine. These might be in people's gardens or growing by the wayside. Whilst he bought in most of the dried herbs and tinctures that he used in his practice, he and Non were also always making tinctures and creams and experimenting with ways of extracting or preserving plants and mushrooms. They seemed to spend more time in their small kitchen mixing up medicines than cooking meals. I was inspired by their willingness to spend time manufacturing a unique single pot of ointment for one patient, whereas in my own practice I would only ever do a large batch in one go.

Chris became well-known for his teaching, first to the general public and then as a clinic supervisor and teacher on professional training courses. By way of charm rather than by self-promotion he came to be seen as something of a sage by many herbalists in the UK and also in the US of A. He tended to share his wisdom not by way of portentous proclamations but by way of quirky anecdotes, understated humour and stories—and this is the side of his teaching revealed in this book. Here we get a glimpse of his gentle teaching style and of his child-like curiosity. He had a knack for helping students understand complex notions by deconstructing them into basic ideas from herbal medicine or physiology. The short sections in this book echo the way he would give lectures—little pieces of information that in themselves sometimes seem whimsical or perhaps insubstantial, but which gradually stack up to reveal inspiring truths.

Non once said to me, "You can tell when Christopher is not in a very good state because he asks the plants for their permission to pick them." She explained that when he was in balance, he was at one with the plants and had no need to ask their consent. The stories and ideas collected in this book perhaps help us readers, too, to become a little more at one with the plants.

bendle, Stoney Middleton
Derbyshire, England
September 2024

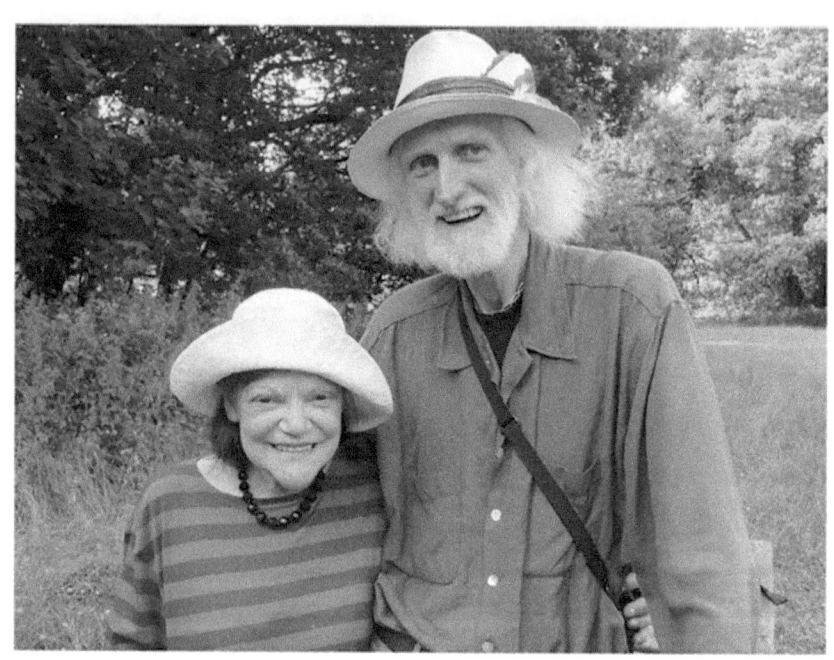
Non Shaw and Christopher Hedley

INTRODUCTION

by Guy Waddell

For my parents, Peter and Yvonne, and my daughters, Minnie and Bea, and their mum, Emma.

"Without doubt she made me what I am today"

Welcome to *Very generous things, plants—we don't deserve them, really*, which is a companion volume to *Plant Medicine: A collection of the teachings of herbalists Christopher Hedley and Non Shaw*[2], and, indeed, to Christopher and Non's *A Herbal Book of Making and Taking*[3]. While *Plant Medicine* contains 500 plus pages of teaching materials developed by Christopher and Non, and *A Herbal Book of Making and Taking* invites you to roll up your sleeves and start making a wide variety of herbal medicines, which is probably more fun than should be allowed in any one book, *Very generous things, plants* is much more personal, compiled from Christopher's spoken words and written communications.

---

[2] Christopher Hedley and Non Shaw, *Plant Medicine—a Collection of the Teachings of Herbalists Christopher Hedley and Non Shaw*, ed. Guy Waddell (London: Aeon Books, 2023).

[3] Christopher Hedley and Non Shaw, *A Herbal Book of Making and Taking* (London: Aeon Books, 2020).

However, just as gentle does not equal weak[4], personal does not equal solipsistic. What is contained in this volume, just like the other two volumes, is based on nearly two lifetimes of learning from plants, herbal medicines, patients, and a long and diverse tradition, all of which are teachers in their own right, and is therefore a reliable source of knowledge that will hopefully be useful in some small or large way to all those with a love of plant medicine. Although Non is not named as an author in this volume, this is simply because she didn't write or speak these words. However, as Christopher said, "Without doubt, she made me what I am today", so Non is undoubtedly here, behind the words and in the spaces and whenever Christopher uses "we", as well as when he doesn't. Christopher and Non both passed away in 2017, with Non departing in the summer and Christopher joining her on the cusp of the autumn equinox. Many people owe their health and direction in life to Christopher and Non, who spent well over sixty years between them in clinical practice and teaching. They were remarkable people who are remembered with love. Please see the introduction to *Plant Medicine* for a reflection on Christopher and Non and their legacy. Of course, in a way, this entire book, being made up of Christopher's words, with Non's presence amongst and behind them, will give you some idea and sense of the people who Christopher and Non were and the rich lives they led.

"Stories are what count"

Christopher loved narratives, seeing them everywhere and recognising their medicinal power, saying, "Stories are what count" and, "Everything is stories". Indeed, Christopher's love of narrative in its many forms, and his use of them as teaching tools, was a key motivation for gathering this collection together. One of the two poets, Ted Kooser and Jim Harrison[5], note in a conversation, that, "Death steals everything except our stories". Similarly, there is a Romany belief[6] that there are two deaths, firstly a material death of the body, and then, hopefully much later, a much more serious second death, when no one can

---

[4] Christopher often referred to Rudolf Weiss's statement that, when it comes to understanding what herbs do, gentle is not the same as weak. See: Rudolf Fritz Weiss, *Herbal Medicine*, 1st ed. (Arcanum, 1988), 1.

[5] Ted Kooser and Jim Harrison, *Braided Creek* (Copper Canyon Press, 2023), 93.

[6] Jan Yoors, *The Gypsies* (Waveland Press, 1987).

remember you anymore. I am sure that Christopher's storytelling will be remembered by all those who knew him, and Christopher and Non will continue to live on for many years to come. I hope this book helps with that endeavour.

"Let's call these people herbalists"

The subtitle to this volume—*Stories, anecdotes and nuggets of wisdom*—indicates that there are various narrative approaches that Christopher uses in his verbal and written communications. In general, *stories* are taken to be narrative journeys with beginnings, middles and ends; *anecdotes* are retellings of events that have happened in the past; and *nuggets of wisdom*, while clearly not an academically accepted term, are somewhat like aphorisms in that they are concisely presented with a value beyond their size, somehow shiny, rather like their gold cousins, and often humorous. Of course, the definitions of these individual categories of narrative can be argued over and anyway they do not have rigid borders between them, but rather leak actively and gently across their membranes to form new ways of narrating worlds. Indeed, stories may be found within Christopher's anecdotes and even in the more pithy nuggets if we look hard enough; anecdotes can be found within the longer stories and as nuggets; and nuggets may be found within stories and anecdotes.

While stories, anecdotes and nuggets loosely describe various forms of narrative, let us briefly consider some terms that might inform our view of the content of this book. "Tales" are often vivid, and this is certainly true of many of Christopher's narratives, which stay with you, resting gently on your shoulders and whispering in your ears over the years. Tales also often include elements of fiction (often mistakenly assumed to be the opposite of "real"), speaking truths that are deeply present and cannot easily be expressed by documented events. A love of folktales is likely to have influenced both the form and content of Christopher's narratives, as you will see. Another term that takes the agency of words one step further and might shed some light on the words between these covers is "imaginal", a term used to suggest the creative power of language as a fundamental part of the abundance of reality[7], as opposed to the imaginary, which points to

---

[7] Tom Cheetham, *Imaginal Love* (Spring Publications, 2015).

the unreal. Imaginal worlds are described as real worlds that can only be accessed via creative imagination[8]. Christopher certainly seemed to bring to life the worlds he described, often mediated by humour, for many of those who heard him speak, and his skills in listening are likely to have been similarly creative for the worlds of his patients. And finally, "pointings" could also be a useful term here, implying something that is being revealed by Christopher but which also requires the reader's own active consideration to bear fruit. Of course, by virtue of its absence from any dictionary, yet also having the quality of being a recognisable term, "pointings" suggests the presence of an accessible magic. Christopher's stories, anecdotes and nuggets of wisdom, or, as we might also call his narratives, tales, imaginal worlds, and pointings, have both truth in them and also often sound and feel magical, much like the man himself. Narratives can create reality and in that sense are a flexible resource for any healer. Truth and the magical walk hand in hand if we relax our vision enough. As Christopher wrote:

> "As far as healing with herbs goes, the story *is* the healing. There exists a class of people whose lives constantly add to these stories—let's call these people herbalists."

While many narratives are driven by degrees of tension and conflict, this is not so with Christopher. Howie Brounstein, an American friend of Christopher's, who you will meet again in this introduction, makes a more than relevant point when he remembers Christopher visiting him one summer. Howie remembers that, "Christopher built a little fairy house out back in the garden. Made of sticks and stones and feathers and such. He said, 'If it stays up for a really long time, the fairies will like it and be happy; if it falls apart quickly, the fairies will be happy and like it.' This is an example of a win-win situation. We don't see these a lot in life." Similarly, Christopher's narratives tend to avoid having "losers", which is probably one reason why, along with their richness, they will draw you back to read them again and again. As if by magic.

---

[8] Marco André Schwarzstein, ed., *Imaginal Worlds* (Thompson, Connecticut : Spring Publications, 2023).

"That'll be 80p"

Christopher's narratives were often humorous, and hopefully they will tickle you too. It is interesting that the only actual "joke" that I remember Christopher telling was a pun. After all, puns often need to be spoken, and in many ways Christopher was part of an (au)(o)ral tradition—listening to the stories told by plants and their interactions with people and then sharing his insights with others. Anyway, here it is, a joke which he also said maybe only Jonathan Treasure, who wrote the foreword to *Plant Medicine*, might understand: "A biochemist walks into a bar and says to the bartender, 'I'll have a pint of adenosine triphosphate, please.' The bartender replies "That'll be 80p." Now, if you're not Jonathan Treasure, it helps if you are a bit of a science geek, or have studied some science and not forgotten it, to get this pun[9].

I am not going to attempt to analyse Christopher's humour here, apart from saying that, unlike "jokes", such as the one above, which are neatly bounded, Christopher's humour was in his bones and in his subtle, understated and often deadpan delivery; in the unexpected examples he gave to illustrate his points; in the way that he gently reduced the complex down to the heart of the matter; in the words he made up but which instantly conveyed their meaning; in the magical stories he told to explain why something might have happened; in the way he turned humour on himself; in the manner in which he anthropomorphised plants without being anthropocentric; in his looking beyond common understandings to gently excavate meanings; in the way that he gave patients, students and herbalists permission to be themselves; and in many other ways that might occur to you as you read this book.

"A criteria of being"

Cornel West[10], the American progressive scholar, activist and 2024 presidential candidate, notes that an important construct in Nietzsche's philosophical imagination was that of a "gay Socrates", which Cornel understands to be a "philosopher who dances", or, "a philosopher with

---

[9] This pun exploits the fact that the "ATP", the acronym of life's energy reservoir "adenosine triphosphate", which was ordered at the bar, is audibly indistinguishable from the cost of a pint of beer in the UK in 1985, with the latter, incidentally and unfortunately, having a net effect in reducing the former.

[10] Cornel West, *Hope on a Tightrope* (Smiley Books, 2008), 41.

a groove". Anyone who has seen Christopher dance will know he had a groove entirely of his own. His grooviness arguably came from his particular combination of an all-encompassing love of living plants and plant medicine, his humour, his openness to the predicaments of his patients as well as his willingness to continue learning from the diverse sources that make up the tradition of herbal medicine. He would not have called himself a philosopher, but as his thinking, which engaged both his brain and his heart, was intimately entangled with plants, it made him a somewhat unique thinker. This could also arguably be seen as being driven by what Hildegard von Bingen (another groovy figure) called *viriditas*, or "greening green",[11] meaning that if Christopher was a stick of Brighton rock, he would be green through and through.

Christopher's green grooviness meant that not only was his practice always busy, but that his teaching sessions, whether at an introductory level, on professional training courses, at Master's level or for practitioners, were always packed full of eager faces, and his herb walks were made up of human planets rotating around Christopher's warm gravity. Christopher's classroom teaching method, for the most part, was to provide comprehensive notes (see *Plant Medicine*) but to put these to one side and tell stories, share anecdotes and provide nuggets of wisdom, even if he would never have called himself wise. He would generally stand up while teaching (although towards the end of a life he did use a tall bar stool to perch on) which made his verticality even more impressive to the class who would usually be seated. The classes would usually be full of laughter and tended to be rather conversational. Arms were always raised. As you will see, he was more than happy to reflect upon and ask questions of the often-intriguing experiences that happen in clinical practice when patients bring their narratives to practitioners. Critical thinking was also part of Christopher's approach, asking whether familiar ideas make sense, if assumptions still hold, and holding both authority and tradition to account, although commonly finding that the latter was the more reliable of the two. Like philosophers, he would also often create new words ("plantocity", or "phlegmatocity") or new concepts ("get below the disease"), as you will see. Crucially, he recognised the need to follow your own path rather than mimic someone else's, saying, "So, we need to have a personal philosophy, a criteria

---

[11] Michael Marder, *Green Mass—the Ecological Theology of St Hildegard of Bingen* (Stanford: Stanford University Press, 2021), 33.

for being (not a justification for action) with an ethos, an inbuilt awareness, and be accepting of responsibility."

"And I was about five ... and I suddenly noticed the Red Deadnettle"

Philosophers, and other academics from anthropologists to political theorists, not surprisingly given the direction of ecological travel in the Anthropocene, are increasingly concerned with the agency of things beyond the human. This includes the developing discipline of vegetal philosophy, which is about fifteen years old, where the ontology and agency of plants are centre stage, after far too long in the academic shadows and undergrowth. While it is difficult to summarise this emergent and rapidly growing field, plants are increasingly seen as being open or unsplit beings, without an inside or outside as we know it, which is particularly attractive for us humans, who experience the separation that having an inside and outside affords. Also, plants are sensitive to their ecologies, indeed merging with them and shifting shape in response to them, and are also without vital organs, think without a head and lead flourishing and generous lives. Overall, they are the sort of critters that suggest the possibility of being different, which is a welcome signal in these troubling times. Given this, while the length of the title to this volume is more of a "nugget" than a story or anecdote, it resonates, in a pithy way (pun intended), with the expansive landscape of vegetal philosophy.[12]

As mentioned, Christopher would never have described himself as a philosopher, and probably hadn't followed the debates in vegetal philosophy. Instead, in many ways, he embodied vegetal philosophy in his actions and interactions, both with plants and with non-sessile critters like you and me. Christopher, through his cultivation of his love of plants, had some of the plant qualities that are described in vegetal philosophy, that we might call "plantabilities". Although, just like you and me, he had an inside and an outside, he also had a quality of openness that was apparent to anyone who spent any time with him. He was

---

[12] Please see the following as a jumping off point to explore some of this terrain: Guy Waddell, "The Matter of Knowing Plant Medicine as Ecology—from Vegetal Philosophy and Plant Science to Tea Tasting in the Anthropocene," in *Plants Matter*, ed. Luci Attala and Louise Steel (Cardiff: University of Wales Press, 2023), 135–59.

sensitive to what he would have called his own "patch", particularly the plants that grew locally to him—indeed, I have seen him merge into a Juniper bush and appear out of nowhere while on a herb walk. He also led a generous life of herbal practice and teaching—while very near to his passing he was giving me instructions on making up and sending out medicines to his patients. And he thought with his heart as much as with his head, including using his intuition (well-earned and grounded in knowledge and experience) as a key part of selecting herbs for his patients, even if he could always justify his choices afterwards. However, he did have vital organs, which eventually gave out. While Christopher's interest in the agency of plants doesn't necessarily make him an accepted philosopher within the academy, it was probably very well received by the plants.

His interest in plants was likely ignited by his father, who would often take him on long walks in the days when kaleidoscopes of butterflies were common encounters. Christopher was undoubtedly a naturalist, even if he didn't have formal qualifications in this discipline, and without this would not have been the herbalist he grew into. His knowledge of living plants, particularly local ones, whether that be between the cracks of pavements, planted in gardens, in parks, on Hampstead Heath, or in London's diminishing wastelands, often drove his knowledge of them as herbal medicines, as we will see. In fact, Christopher remembers the following:

> "I was about five ... and I suddenly noticed the Red Deadnettle, I think that was the first individual plant that I noticed. I think that, at that moment the fairies planted the seed in my soul, maybe they did it earlier, I don't know, but that's the moment I remember."

Christopher's own plant-ness undoubtedly grew out of his very close relationships with these plants in his patch. His observations of, and participations with, plants, then acted as a compost to develop his ideas around what plants may actually be doing in a body.

"How the plant is in the world, is how it will be in your body"

The doctrine of signatures, which was developed by Paracelsus in the Middle Ages, but had precedent in the work of Pliny the Elder and Dioscorides, was a doctrine that attributed medicinal properties to plants based on their particular features, including colour, shape, texture and smell. For example, the yellow colour of Greater Celandine reveals an attribution to cure liver ailments; the appearance of Eyebright indicates its appropriation to the eyes; plants that grow in stony environments point to the breaking up of renal calculi; and Pine seeds that resemble teeth indicate the leaves should be boiled in water and taken for toothache. Moderns mostly discredit the doctrine of signatures, for example, seeing it as an a priori clue to therapeutic value, arguing that it should rather be seen as a mnemonic, a way of remembering therapeutic value[13]. Whatever you think of this, it is interesting that the doctrine's focus tends to be limited to plant appearance and anatomy rather than to anything more connected to its environment. In the latter stages of his life, Christopher noted that, "How the plant is in the world, is how it will be in your body", indicating that it might be fruitful to extend this association between plants and their therapeutic interactions with people from their appearance to how plants *are* and what plants *do* in their ecologies. For example, you will find, in this book, that Astragalus root, as a member of the pea family, "strengthens the ground in which they grow", so Astragalus as a medicine, "holds things, good and bad", pointing towards its traditional contraindication in acute infections. Water figwort (*Scrophularia aquatica*), a "marshy plant ... spreads by rhizomes, creeping along as the land dries. We use this mainly for lymphatic congestion with heavy water retention in the lower body." And, Golden Seal's habit of spreading just below the surface indicates its medicinal use for "solidifying surfaces". This shift in focus from plant structure in the doctrine of signatures to plant ecologies in Christopher's thinking might be named the doctrine of plant behaviours. Of course, doctrine sounds rather dogmatic and unflexible to modern ears, especially given its association with religion, politics and warfare, and also inflexible to those who are aware of Christopher's desire to avoid authoritarianism and singularity in herbal medicine, preferring pluralism and the importance of finding your own way of practicing. However, the origin of "doctrine" is from Latin "doctrina" meaning "teaching, learning", with the medical meaning only arising in the 14th century, so we'll stick with this word as a way of contributing

---

[13] Bradley C Bennett, "Doctrine of Signatures: Through Two Millennia," *HerbalGram*, no. 78 (2008): 34–45, https://www.herbalgram.org/resources/herbalgram/issues/78/table-of-contents/article3244/.

in some way to reclaiming the original meaning. Of course, there is the question as to whether, if this doctrine holds water, it has to hold true for all medicinal plants, and also whether it is an *aide memoire* or a way of learning from nature. I shall leave readers to make their own minds up on this. Maybe you can add to the story.

"Traditional roots and phytochemical branches"

Christopher reflected that his Physiomedical teachers used complex formulae of up to forty herbs in a prescription. Christopher, however, noted that:

> "(I was) drawn to herbal medicine by the plants themselves … No one told me that I could learn directly from the plants themselves—although the concept lurked in my mind as it seemed intrinsic to Culpeper's method and he was my original inspiration. Culpeper liked simples and the constituent chemistry people went for simple formulae. Thus, I evolved a system with traditional roots and phytochemical branches—and have spent the next twenty odd years trying to find a trunk."

One way of approaching this trunk, that I hope Christopher would approve of, is to look at how phytochemistry might meet vegetal philosophy, as encountered earlier, as well as recent plant science. Phytochemically speaking, while primary plant metabolites (such as amino acids, carbohydrates, and vitamins) are directly required for the growth and development of plants, it is the secondary plant metabolites (such as phenolics, alkaloids, saponins, and terpenes) that are mostly responsible for both the medicinal properties of plants as well as for mediating plant-environment interactions. Interestingly, just as philosophy has engaged in new ways with plants over recent times, a new direction of research within plant sciences has also made quite radical— perhaps that should be "radicle"—leaps over the last twenty-five years or so. While plant science has long argued that secondary plant metabolites generally provide defence against pests and pathogens, protection against UV radiation and stress, and release attractive volatile compounds, it is the relatively recent developments within plant science that have moved the focus to plant behaviour and plant intelligence, concepts that were previously inconceivable in the rather conservative botanical sciences. These developments have demonstrated that plants can forage for nutrients and water, select the most viable source, are aware of whether other plants or inanimate objects are producing shade near them, have a sensitivity to touch which includes the ability to avoid touching each other's crowns ("crown shyness"), are able to recognise plant kin through their interactions and gestures, can decide to share available resources with their kin and make exchanges with others, as well as anticipate reward and learn what is dangerous or not.[14]

It seems reasonable to suggest that, at a phytochemical level, it is the diverse realm of secondary plant metabolites that, as well as providing medicines for humans, mostly allows and facilitates, or even drives, depending on the degree of agency that we give to phytochemical matter, the "plantabilities" emerging from both plant science and vegetal philosophy. Given this, and if we accept that plants' lack of an inside and outside makes them open beings that have no boundaries with their ecologies, so that essentially, they *are* ecology, then maybe the simple truth of the (plant) matter is that the benefits of ingesting plant medicines are arrived at through us becoming less separate, even nonseparate, from our ecology, which is now no longer outside of us, but of which we are part. Whole may be synonymous with healed, might be one way of putting it.

Of course, this brings us back to Christopher's "traditional roots", because traditional peoples have always had such an understanding of their place in and of the world. Whether we start with plant chemistry, vegetal philosophy or new plant science, we end up at the place occupied by traditional knowledge, which was always Christopher's most reliable and beloved knowledge source.

I wonder what phytochemical messages were travelling within and between plants and Christopher when they encountered him on a herb walk. Maybe this has something to do with how well-loved his herb walks were. I suspect that Christopher may have produced the odd secondary plant metabolite of his own, ultimately helping his patients to feel less separate and more whole, taking the consultation home with them in the bottles and bags and jars of herbs that had been dispensed for them and from which he and his love of plants were inseparable.

---

[14] Waddell, *The Matter of Knowing Plant Medicine as Ecology*.

The book to come

An irony in editing this book is that, in dividing it up into various thematic parts (history, *materia medica*, and living plants and philosophy of practice), Christopher's narratives have been "sectored-and-scissored" to borrow a phrase from Ronald Grimes[15]. However, while reading this book might not be quite like sitting in the same room as Christopher, or being on the welcome receiving end of his electronic words, it is hoped that you get a flavour of Christopher. A sip, slurp or glug, at least. Only minor edits have been made for clarity, so it should be clear which texts were spoken and which were written.

The names of the three parts of this book are similarly found in *Plant Medicine*, which is worth describing here. In *Plant Medicine*, *Part 1 Roots* feels its way down into the soil of historical knowledge as a foundation for plant medicine; *Part 2 Flowers*—named such because it is often medicinal plant knowledge that attracts people to herbal medicine in the first place, rather like pollinators to flowers—focuses on the materia medica that Christopher and Non found so useful; *Part 3 Fruits* is concerned with herbal therapeutics, arguably the sweet reward of applying materia medica knowledge for the benefit of people in need of help; and *Part 4 Seeds* looks at some of the key threads of Christopher and Non's practices, going within to look at tea tasting and the minutiae of plant chemistry, and going beyond in its engagement with Chinese medicine and the value of examining plant families as a way of understanding medicinal plants. As such, *Part 4 Seeds*, like its botanical namesake, is full of potential in its exploration of key elements of herbal practice.

In *Very generous things, plants,* as similar a line as possible has been taken, although in the volume you hold in your hands, *Fruits* are missing, with this being because Christopher rarely spoke about particular conditions in his recorded teachings and email communications, preferring to focus on physiology and traditional knowledge when working out ways of treating people. So, in this volume, *Roots* is concerned solely with humoral medicine, unlike *Plant Medicine* which included Physiomedicalism. Of course, other traditions are addressed elsewhere in this book, notably in *Seeds*. *Roots* is followed by *Flowers*, and, similarly

---

[15] Ronald Grimes, "Performance Is Currency in the Deep World's Gift Economy: An Incantatory Riff for a Global Medicine Show," in *The Handbook of Contemporary Animism*, ed. Graham Harvey (London: Routledge, 2013), 506. Readers might like to check out this book for some perspectives that resonate with Christopher's way of being with plants.

to *Plant Medicine*, focuses on materia medica, the irresistible centre of herbal medicine. *Seeds* is slightly different here, with the focus being on the living plants themselves and on philosophy of practice, with these two being deeply entangled, of course. Hopefully the interconnectedness between the two volumes makes them truly complementary companion volumes of each other. Maybe they'll keep each other company on your bookshelves.

So, to give a little more detail about this volume, the focus of *Roots—Resourcing humoral thinking for plant medicine* is humoral medicine, specifically Galenic humoral medicine, the application of which to clinical practice was a central part of Christopher's story as a herbalist. It was Galen, born in 129 CE, who reworked the somewhat loose and baggy humoral medicine of the Hippocratic school, from around 400 BCE, into a tighter, and some would argue, even rigid, discipline of medicine, which persisted as the dominant medical system in Europe until the 17th century. While Galen was the originator of this approach, it was Nicholas Culpeper's no-nonsense yet open sensibility and engagement with this tradition that resonated most closely with Christopher, and which can be felt most clearly in the following stories, anecdotes and nuggets of wisdom. Just as Galen breathed fresh air into the Hippocratic tradition, and Culpeper arguably did the same with the Galenic tradition that was getting a bit stale, so Christopher has taken up and run with this tradition, ensuring its relevance for today's patients. This part is divided up into five sections, namely the four individual humours considered one by one, followed by a consideration of the four humours together[16].

While *Roots* highlights that Christopher was in some ways a practitioner in the humoral tradition, although not limited by it, the focus of *Flowers—Materia medica of plant medicine* reveals that Christopher drew on a diverse number of herbal threads when discussing the herbal medicines that he loved so much. These include the plants themselves; traditional knowledge—particularly humoral medicine, especially of Culpeper, and Physiomedical and Eclectic practitioners; clinical experience (his and others'); folk knowledge; and orthodox physiology,

---

[16] Please see *Plant Medicine* for a more detailed consideration of Galenic humoral medicine, as well as the wider history of herbal medicine, including Physiomedicalism, and for further reading.

preferring that as a basis for practice much more than pathophysiology, as well other sciences.

Seeds—Living plants and philosophy of practice for plant medicine reflects the later stages of Christopher's professional life. While he still found much value in Galenic humoral theory, he was more concerned with herbal energetics. He did not regard energetics as knowing the degrees of hot, cold, damp and dry of medicinal plants, rather he understood this to mean getting to know the herb directly, especially spending time with the living plants that provide themselves as medicine. He was, after all, a naturalist as much as a herbalist. In fact, throughout this book you can see how knowledge of living plants informs his practice, even if it is more of a focus in *Seeds*. Of course, many herbalists feel this way—that not only do living herbs nourish herbalists' lives but they also inform their practices, but Christopher somehow gave permission to many herbalists to allow this relationship to become central in their lives.

Acknowledgements

There are a lot of people to thank for making this book possible. Firstly, thank you to Christopher's brother David for permission to publish Christopher's spoken words and written communications, and Tina Harvey, Non's sister, for permission to use Non's artwork so skilfully and respectfully used in the book design by Phil Deakin, as he did in *Plant Medicine*. Thank you, all! And a big thank you to bendle, a close friend and colleague of Christopher's, for his foreword to this volume. You might also like to see "Up until that point" in *Seeds*, for a lesson that bendle taught Christopher.

I would like to reserve a very special thank you to Howie Brounstein, a friend of Christopher's, who you met above in his story about the fairy house. Howie is a herbalist, botanist, wildcrafter and educator at Columbines School of Botanica Studies and, very importantly for the genesis of this book, the administrator of Herbal Hall, a US-based, but international, internet discussion group for professional herbalists, where Christopher felt at home between 1999 and 2017. Many thanks to him for permission to include Christopher's email posts. Without this source material, you would be enjoying much thinner soup—*Flowers* and *Seeds* would be especially diminished. Thank you, Howie! I would also like to thank Matthew Seal for making such accurate notes at a

London teaching of Christopher's, enabling the title to this volume to be arrived at, and to Cristina Cromer for her crystal-clear memory of a conversation with Christopher.

I would now like to thank a number of people for permission to use recordings of Christopher's teaching as source material for this volume. First of all, thank you to Robyn Soma, president of the National Institute of Medical Herbalists (NIMH), for permission to use a recording of a talk called "Roots and Branches" that Christopher gave at the 2013 NIMH conference and AGM. Also, thank you to Nathalie Chidley for permission to use a recording of Christopher teaching Galenic humoral medicine that she made in 2012 at the University of Middlesex. And to Jay and Bridget Johnson, of Tree Farm Communications, for permission to use the following recordings of Christopher's teachings in the USA in 2000 at the Pacific Northwest Herbal Symposium, namely on the subjects of "Treating Heart and Circulatory Diseases in Elders", "Traditional European Herbs for Maintaining a Long and Healthy Life", and "The Galenic Humoral System in Practice and How it Can Help Maintain Optimum Health", and, in 2011 at the 10th International Herb Symposium for permission to use recordings on the subjects "A Taste of Herbs", "A Story of Herbs", and "From Birth to Death—How the Galenic Humoral System Looks at Life". Please check out their website for these recordings and further treats.[17]

Of course, the book wouldn't have been possible at all without Oliver Rathbone, a herbalist who, luckily for herbal medicine, also happens to be a publisher. A rare breed indeed! Without Oliver and Alice Rathbone, and their stewardship at Aeon books, along with Eve Brazil's attention to detail, Christopher and Non's teachings would have likely taken much longer to be turned into the pleasure of turning pages, or scrolling in an ebook. Thank you! And thank you so much to Liz Oldham, who taught alongside Christopher and myself at the University of Westminster, for a close reading of the draft text, identifying much needed corrections.

I would also like to thank Nick Pearson, a psychotherapist whose knowledge and love of Sufism and the role of the imagination in healing is a central part of his work with his clients. I have learnt from Nick the value of helping clients to cultivate that subtle place of awareness—which is entirely separate from thought—which they then bring to the predicament of their own bodies. This may result in images arising,

---

[17] Tree Farm Communications. 2025. https://treefarmtapes.com/

similarly to pertinent dream images and other images that suitably resonate, which clients can engage with in emotionally powerful and potentially transformative ways for both lives and the bodies that live them. As Rumi[18] said:

> But don't be satisfied with stories, how things
> have gone with others. Unfold
> your own myth, without complicated explanations,
> so everyone will understand the passage,
> *We have opened you.*

And, of course, Christopher has opened many to new possibilities through the world of plants, the medicines made from them and his patients' narratives gently decocted down during time spent with him to reveal insights that guide them on their way.

I would especially like to thank my daughters, Minnie and Bea, and their mum, Emma, an artist, for persevering while I worked on this volume, while they have been working on their own creations. And my parents, Peter and Yvonne, for constantly surprising me with their humour and resilience, and my devilishly handsome twin brother, Mark, and his wife and son, Emily and Huxley, for being themselves.

Disclaimer

This book is not intended to be a substitute for appropriate medical care from a healthcare practitioner. If you, or someone you know, needs help, seek it out from a qualified healthcare practitioner.

---

[18] Rumi, *Selected Poems*, trans. Coleman Barks et al. (London: Penguin, 2004), 41.

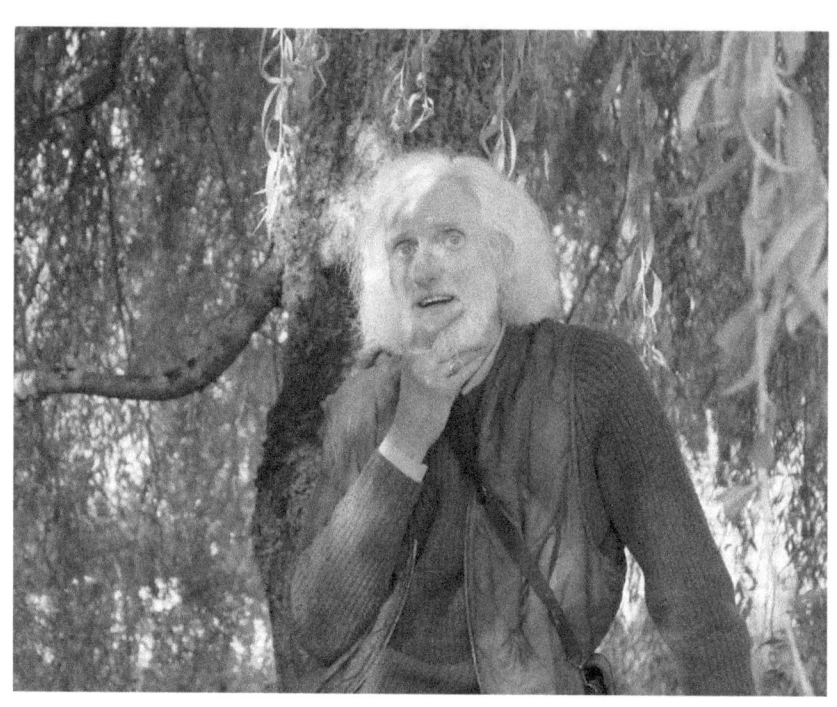

Photo by Amanda Cook

Roots—Resourcing Humoral Thinking for Plant Medicine

The Choleric Humour

They'll get up and walk out

So, the first type, we've got to do the choleric type first. The first type is the fire type, the choleric type. If we don't do them first, they'll get up and walk out. So, the choleric humour is what you get in a person when fire is manifested in that person. Fire people tend to be short. The saying is that fire gives form. Culpeper has a nice way of saying it. He says fire burns up all the air, so fiery people are very compact. Compact is probably better than short, probably better, but they tend on the whole to be short. So, if you think of a fairly short, muscular, bouncy, aggressive person, perhaps with red hair, then you know a fiery person, don't you? You probably know somebody like that.

They have a very direct gaze. Fire is expressed in the eyes a lot. So, a fiery person tends to look straight at you. Has a very direct gaze. Everyone else is a bit shifty, aren't they? I don't see many purely choleric people in my practice, because I don't have an accident and emergency department. Mostly you'll only see choleric people when they have an accident. When they fall off a mountain or smash their sports car or whatever, that's when you mostly see them. Sometimes they get really, really ill and they allow themselves to worry a little about it and they'll come to see you and they're the most godawful patients, honestly. They are dreadful. They don't do anything they're told.

So, how do we do it? How do we get through to them? Fiery people appreciate directness. So, you'd be very direct and straight. They appreciate discipline. They like discipline. If you want to get fiery people to exercise more, then you have to engage their fieriness in it. You have to say, "I know, why don't you go out one day and play squash?" That's a good one, isn't it? You can easily get fiery people engaged in playing squash. Fiery people like short, easily attainable goals. That's what they like. It's no good saying to them, look, getting better takes a long time, you have to change, you have to do this and that, because they've gone out the door by then. You have to give them short, easily attainable goals. You have to say, "I know, let's do a three day fast. Well, let *you* do a three day fast."

It just came out

A friend of ours is very fire and water, and for a long time I never saw his fire at all. I always thought he was phlegmatic and watery. He was quite soft and quiet. He was very submissive to his partner and I don't know, anyway, but he worked as a psychotherapist with teenagers, which does require fire, so the fire must have been there. Then his mother got a brain tumour and died, and he was a single; he wasn't a single parent, she was a single parent, if you see what I mean. His father had run off when he was a child. He started suffering all sorts of different complaints. His fire came up and he started suffering abscesses and fiery things. Especially fiery and watery things, to do with an abscess. Basically, abscesses and boils and things like that. And talking to him, it was ever so interesting because what happens when you start talking about fire and water with him, he starts putting together the ideas in his head. When he was a teenager and his fire was coming up, he deliberately suppressed it, because his mother would worry about him. So, he suppressed his fire completely and hid it and when his mother died, it just came out. It was amazing to watch, and so I said, "Well now you're going to have learn how to be fiery all over again, aren't you?" So, he used to like going to Barcelona for holidays. So, I said, "What you do, you go to Barcelona, you find a nice macho fiery Spanish man walking down the street and you follow him, make sure he doesn't see, and adjust your posture." If you walk in a fiery way it'll bring out your fiery things. So just follow him, and yeah, be walking in a fiery way.

It's tough

As you're going through life, what happens is you start off warm and wet, as you go through life you start to dry out. As you go through life from infant to older and to elder, so your vitality goes down, and your dampness go down and you start to dry out. So, summer is warm and dry and it's the time of adolescence. The time of fertility or at least the things that might lead to fertility. Like wearing very few clothes. The heat remains high, but we dry out, we enter adolescence, the choleric stage, but adolescents still tend to retain some of the old patterns of childhood. So, they have plenty of vitality but not as much as they did have when they were younger. So, they tend to burn it all up very quickly and then not get out of bed 'til three days later—that's a sort of typical adolescent pattern. It's a very difficult time, isn't it, adolescence, do you remember? Tough, it was. It's hard.

Move your body

This happens a lot to students, I see it a lot in my choleric students. What choleric people must be doing is they must be moving their body, it's very, very important; the fire tissue in the body is the muscles. They need to exercise those muscles and keep them moving, it's extremely important. The last thing a fiery person should do is sit down and study. Sitting down is bad for us, no activity, and studying is thinking too much. So, when you bump into fiery students towards the end of the course, they're often quite depressed and you say, "Well, when did you last exercise?" "Oh", they say, "Oh, I haven't got time to exercise, I've got to study." And you say, "Last night you sat down, you looked at that book and you read through the page and you got to the end of the page and you'd forgotten what was at the beginning. And then you have to read it all over again, and it's wasting your time. Go out and exercise, come home, read the page and it'll make perfect sense." It works really, really well. You have to nourish and look after your different humours.

Do you want a recipe?

There's a famous 18th Century treatment for that. They say if the fire dies out because it's suppressed, you're not basically nourishing it—it dies out and leaves ashes. And the ashes are quite light, and they accumulate at the top part of the body. And you get what they call "burnt choler", which is a type of melancholy. So, when you say melancholy affects the heart, you actually mean suppressed fire, basically. So, it's depression in the heart. This can happen to students who stop doing other things to study and to elders when they retire and stop doing their doing thing. Do you want a recipe? The recipe is Motherwort, Borage and Lemon Balm[1]. They're three herbs which work well together to clear poisons from the heart, basically, and protect the heart.

Introduce the idea

Sometimes the healing is done just by talking about things, actually. I was talking to a woman the other day, and I just thought, she was very obviously a very fiery, choleric person and she was confused. And I just pointed out, I just introduced the idea of fieriness slowly into the conversation and pointed out that that was her main characteristic and what the implications were, and she just burst into tears. It was amazing. We could probably do without the herbs or the homeopathy or whatever, couldn't we? Just helping people to understand themselves.

Just pretend

Ok, relating to fiery people: if you've got a fiery patient, do not back away. The fiery person will sit there and look at you and sit forward. Under no circumstances back away, otherwise they just keep coming. Just pretend you're fiery.

---

[1] I suspect Christopher came across this recipe at the Wellcome library in London. Culpeper's comments on the individual uses of these herbs certainly supports the idea that they might be used together like this. See: Nicholas Culpeper, *Culpeper's Complete Herbal* (1653; repr., Wordsworth Reference, 1995). The use of this combination is echoed by Stephen Taylor in his recent book. See: Stephen Taylor, *The Humoral Herbal* (Aeon Books, 2021), 160. Perhaps of interest is that, in *The Anatomy of Melancholy*, published a year before *Culpeper's Complete Herbal*, Burton points out that the physician Crato, when considering the treatment of melancholy caused by black choler, "speaks against all herbs and worts, except borage, bugloss, fennel, parsley, dill, balm, succory", suggesting that, for Burton at least, Lemon Balm and Borage may be of benefit. There is no mention of Motherwort, though. See: Robert Burton, *The Anatomy of Melancholy* (1652; repr., London: Chatto and Windus, 1883), 189. https://www.exclassics.com/anatomy/anatomy1.pdf. [Ed.]

Scattered fire

In the Hippocratic tradition every element should be in its place. If the fire is suppressed, it will move and scatter and do things it shouldn't be doing. You'll be getting fire in different parts of the body doing things it shouldn't be doing. So, for example, what I always think of as scattered fire, the first thing it tends to do is rise. If it rises to the head, then you get anger. Anger can be useful activity, even if it does involve shooting the neighbours because at least you get some satisfaction from doing that. If it rises to the heart, then you get mania, which is basically activity which is not useful—you're just rushing around, not doing anything particular, spending everybody's money and, like one of my patients, discovering the meaning, the meaning of life and how to cure everybody, which in her opinion was pogo sticks. She actually wrote a letter to Prince Charles saying that everybody would be better if they used pogo sticks everyday. Well, I don't think he replied himself, but she got a reply.

Really strong and solid in the centre

Fire brings light, of course, and clarity. Fiery people are always very quick at picking up ideas. You need a little bit of fire in your brain. So, without the fire going to the brain, you get a lack of concentration. If the fire goes to other parts of your body and gets scattered over your body, you get aches and pains, especially sharp, stabbing pains and you'll get periods of feeling hot and cold, especially when you go to bed and people will say, "I think I'm menopausal, even though I'm only twenty-eight, because I get really hot at night", but it's nothing to do with that, it's just to do with the fire not being held in its place. So, you get the fire type of insomnia which is hyper-alertness, not worrying but just not being able to get to sleep because your fire's looking for something to do all the time. The best remedies for excess fire or scattered fire or fire out of its place are bitters. And the reason bitters are good is because they consolidate, they bring you to the centre. One of my favourite terms from Chinese medicine is that bitters are consolidating. You know the taste of bitters, you know that nice, satisfying, "I feel really strong and solid in the centre" feeling. As the bitters sink, of course, they pull the heat down and return it to its place. That's the reason why bitters are so good in digestion, because they sink, which, therefore, can improve the flow of food through the digestive tract. Down and out.

Two tissues

Choleric people generally need cooling herbs because they get hot and overheat. The two tissues in the body which produce most heat are the muscles, and choleric people tend to be quite muscular, and the liver of course, because the liver does the great load of the metabolic processes in the body, so therefore the liver tends to overproduce heat. So, I always like to say to students, put your hand over your liver and then put your hand over your stomach. You find your liver's usually running noticeably warmer. It's all that metabolism going on in there, isn't it?

Jump off mountains

Ok. So, most people don't fit clearly into one category. We're all ratios, aren't we? One of the useful things about treating sick people rather than healthy people, is that in sick people one humour tends to dominate. If you've got two dominant humours then usually you would get sick along one of those humours, not along both at the same time. It's a bit tricky to do that. The basis of humoral pathology is that we always play to our strengths. Fiery people always do fiery things, they always jump off mountains and whatever and drive fast cars and such.

But then it's over

They're really clear thinkers, they'll go straight to the point. It might not be the most important point but it's a point. And at their worst they're angry and irritable, bitter. But I always say, if you're going to upset somebody, if you're going to upset someone always upset a choleric person because they respond straightaway. You might get a good kicking but then it's over and they may even become your best friend.

The Sanguine Humour

Extra bouncy

The time when everybody is at least a little bit sanguine is in childhood. And, obviously if you're a sanguine child, then you're even more sanguine, extra bouncy. Sanguine is the air humour, it has a lot of movement in it. You can tell that with children, you see them walking down the street to school and they're skipping, skippety-skip and they have to run forwards and backwards to their mother, don't they, because it's compulsory. My very first memory is running round the home where my parents lived, just running round, just for the sheer joy of running.

New things

The reason why, of course, children are airy, is because that's what they've got to do, they've got to be interested in new things. That's what children have got to be. They've got to be constantly picking up ideas and assembling them. That's the time of learning in life.

Talking airy people into getting better

So, the way you deal with sanguine people, with airy people, is the same as the way you treat small children—you're authoritative. Children love authority, don't they? Children like their parents to know everything and life becomes difficult when you suddenly realise they don't know everything and so life starts to trip you up. So, if you're treating airy patients, it's all you have to do. You can often talk them into getting better, just by being authoritative. It's quite useful to have done all the physiology and pathology, which you probably cursed at the time, because then you can talk the language that the medical profession talk and they'll come along with that and if you can drop those long words every now and then into the sentence, doesn't really matter where they fit, as long as they're dropped in, then, that gives the airy person's confidence in you and they'll just get better just because they have confidence in you.

Air settles eventually

Through your whole life, try and keep in touch with all your humours to some extent and don't try and rely too much on one strategy all the time. They do say, I'm looking forward to this, they do say of sanguine people, of airy people, that the older they get the better they get because the air will settle. I'm looking forward to that.

Just like that

They like flirting and foreplay. The head, the head can be full of unquiet thoughts. That's a good phrase, isn't it? "Unquiet thoughts". They tend to see an accumulation of heat and damp, which tends to ulcers and abscesses and boils and things of that kind. I had a patient once, he was very, very airy and he was a croupier in a gambling casino, which is probably not a good idea really, because apart from anything else, airy people tend to have no good fixed habits. They tend to be scattered, scattered, scattered and one of the first things to do with airy people suffering from airy things is to say, I want you to have fixed habits. I usually say three meals a day, whatever the circumstances are, eat three meals a day: boom, boom, boom. So, that's the focus for the rest of your day. Of course, you're not doing that if you're working late in the evening and things like that. He was covered in boils. Then, I just gave him Marigold, because of what we do anyway, but just talked to him about airiness. He gave up the job, actually, and went and lived on a remote Scottish isle and became a smallholder. Pretty extreme, isn't it? I don't know how he's doing, haven't spoken to him since. But they can do that, just move on, bish, bash, bosh, just like that.

Catapults in the front room

In the Greek understanding, in fact, we say "Galenic" because Galen was the chap who wrote it all down. Galen was a Roman army doctor originally, so you can imagine what sort of a pain he was to live with, probably putting up those catapults in the front room or something. He just wrote it all down, unlike others. Therefore, he's right, at least it's easy to say he's right. So, we call it Galenic or Greek anyway. In this system, air is hot and wet. So, you mustn't get it mixed with the Ayurvedic air system, which is different because they're in a different country. So, in Greece the air is hot and wet. So, sanguine people tend to be hot and wet. The physical attribute of the body, which is most hot and wet, of course, is the blood. So, sanguine people are regarded as full blooded. They're quite often red, at least in white people. Falstaff, I think, in Shakespeare, is a very typical sanguine person. A great joy for life, a great lust for life. "Wine, women and song", or "wine, men and song", or "wine, person and song", or whatever your flavour is, more or less sums it up, I suppose.

Sanguinosity

My favourite illustration of sanguine patients is a patient I had a few years ago, he was an opera singer. Can you beat that? OK. So, what always strikes me when I go to the opera is the price of the shoes. All the money they spend on the costumes! It's sanguinosity. A lot of sanguinosity around the opera. He is an opera singer and he was basically quite healthy but he had, like a lot of airy people, an unbalanced circulation. Because air is shifting, flowing, shifting, flowing, so the circulation is unbalanced. In a fiery person the circulation is always right there on top. In an airy person it comes and goes. So, he had varicose ulcers, because the blood wasn't flowing properly, so we gave him some treatment. Gave him some Comfrey ointment and some medications and things. We went into his lifestyle, and we said, "What do you eat?" He said, "Three or four bottles of wine." "No, what do you eat?", we said. Basically, he didn't eat at home at all. He always went out. He'd be eating very late. He'd be going to the opera performing and then going out with friends and the cast and things like that, having very rich food, lots of bottles of wine and it was, that's a typical sanguine thing to do, to overindulge yourself in rich things. The time of your life where we're most sanguine is when we're babies. So, sanguine people are like babies. They like rich food, they like to be indulged, they like the company of women or men. So, they tend to overindulge themselves. So, we said, "OK, we'll give you a regime", and we worked out a regime. It's always a matter of negotiation, isn't it? Negotiated a regime with him, which was sort of eating reasonable food, not eating too late and so on and so forth. After two or three months, all his ulcers were better, he was fine. No trouble at all. A couple of months later he came back and they'd all come back again and we said, "What's happened?" So, he said, "I couldn't do that, you know, I just couldn't keep that up. I've got to see my friends. If I see my friends I've got to go out to the restaurant. If I go out to restaurants, it's got to be a good restaurant. It's a French restaurant where there's lashings of cream and sugar and they'd all come back again." We said, "Well, you know what to do." He said, "Yes, but I'm not going to do it. It's not worth it. I'd rather have the ulcers", and that was the last we saw of him.

The only person to cycle up that hill

I had a patient who was, I still have this patient actually, I see him every now and then. It's a different thing each time he comes. He's incredibly fit. He's the only person I know that cycles up, what's that big hill? Muswell Hill. He cycles up Muswell Hill![2] I saw him once, he had

---

[2] For those of you who like numbers, Muswell Hill is 0.6 km long, ascends by 56 m and has an average gradient of 8.8%. At least if you cycle up it, you might have an opportunity to cycle down as well. [Ed.]

really nasty cystitis because he cycled to South of France and back in a weekend. He's fit. In a weekend, well, maybe it's a long weekend. He is seriously fit. He came because his granny died of a heart attack and he started worrying about his heart and blood pressure. When I took it, his blood pressure would go up as you were taking it. His blood pressure was obviously quite fine, he was terrified, and you took it and it would go up as you were taking it, you know. In the end his GP was very clever, he sent him to see a special blood pressure psychotherapist, and this blood pressure psychotherapist said, "OK, I'm going to put this cuff on your arm now and then we're going to talk about something else", and they'd take a blood pressure, then they'd talk about something else and then take his blood pressure. Just desensitising basically to blood pressure taking and his blood pressure turned out to be all right. And then he comes with something else. It's a really good idea to see patients' bodies, isn't it, so you can see what's going on. When he takes his clothes off, he's all massive tension, tension, tension, tension, tension, and then this big knot there and he acknowledges that. Gave him Gentian and Chamomile to settle, because Chamomile appropriates to the solar plexus, but Chamomile doesn't really have any much direction to it, so add Gentian to give the direction, works really, really, really well. Chamomile and Gentian just to get that, the energy moving down to his body, to his lower body, instead of being up here in his head all the time.

Began to eat

The best sanguine people are childlike, at worst they're childish. Childlike—full of wonder, generous, always interested in new ideas, loving company, good food, singing. Or childish—easily bored, fickle, restless, disorganised, unfaithful, prone to hypochondria and an erratic lifestyle. My favourite Galenic constitutional primer is Winnie the Pooh, I highly recommend that you read Winnie the Pooh if you're interested in this whole subject. So, which of the main characters in Winnie the Pooh, do you think, has the most sanguine disposition? Winnie the Pooh, absolutely! Tends to be a bit self-indulgent, everybody loves them and, like children, they've only got to smile, and everybody loves you! They tend to be self-indulgent, they like eating rich food and they get stuck down rabbit holes because they've eaten all the honey. It is a very, very good book actually, it's very useful. I've got a quote, "'Piglet', said Pooh solemnly, 'what shall we do?' And he began to eat

Tigger's sandwiches." Children and sanguine adults should avoid sweet food, or they will get stuck in the rabbit hole. They should avoid concentrated, sweet and warming and damp foods. Refined sugar is the worst. I suppose we're quite lucky that Pooh didn't have sugar, he just had honey which isn't quite so bad. When I was a child, my mother used to give me, as a special treat, white bread spread with margarine and sprinkled with white sugar, it's a wonder I'm still alive, isn't it?

Turmeric hair

So, what else about airy people? Yes, herbs to calm. Valerian is very good. Skullcap, Passion Flower, all those obvious ones, and Turmeric. I quite like Turmeric. Turmeric is a very useful herb for overcoming blockages, emotional blockages. Sort of gentle and warm. I once went for a massage with a Tibetan who was training with an acupuncturist, and he used lots of infused oils for massage, and he obviously sussed me out, thinking, "He's a very airy person", and massaged me with Turmeric infused oil. It was quite nice. It was a nice massage. I went and looked in the mirror afterward and I was totally covered in yellow and I washed as much off my hands and face as best as I could to go back on the Tube. People kept looking at me, which does happen a lot anyway, but people kept looking at me and I got home and my hair was bright yellow. Good massage though. Smoothed out the blockages.

The Phlegmatic Humour

Fluxions of rheum

The word "rheumatism" originally meant "fluxions of rheum",[3] meaning excess phlegm from the head. In traditional medicine, the head was regarded to be full of phlegm, probably still is, isn't it? Because if you cut the brain open, of course, it's obviously phlegmy, isn't it? It's soggy. And the phlegm would sometimes overflow, it would overflow in one of two directions. It would come out your nose and people would say, "Ah right, there's the phlegm overflowing." And the other thing is it

---

[3] After the waning of the dominance of Galenic medical thinking, "rheumatism" came to be viewed as a painful "fluxion", meaning movement of tissues between the skin and internal organs, before modern scientific understandings of rheumatism as a group of inflammatory disorders affecting connective tissues gained ascendency. [Ed.]

went down the inside. It would come down the inside and settle in the muscles. And phlegm being cold and wet would then cause contraction and stiffness in the muscle and you'd get general aches and pains, of the sort that my grandfather used to say, "it's going to rain tomorrow, my right arm aches."

Cheese and pepper

Phlegmatic people should avoid all cold and wet foods, such as milk. They're the people who mustn't have milk because if they have milk, they're immediately blocked and clogged up, like a lot of us are, but particularly phlegmatic people. They must avoid cold foods and they must always have a bit of spice with their food. One of my all-time favourites in Ayurvedic medicine is a "Ayurveda: The Science of Self-Healing"[4] by Dr Lad and the reason I like it is because on the back page it says what to add to your foods to balance them. I thought that was good. I thought, right I can have cheese if I have lots of pepper with it. Great, I like this man.

Damn, I've had my leg shot off

Phlegm is the watery humour. If water is high in a person, we call that person phlegmatic. Water is cold and wet. Classically speaking, the English are supposed to be phlegmatic. You've probably used the expression "phlegmatic." It's still used in common parlance, isn't it? Who is the, I can't think of his name now, the guy that stood next to the Duke of Wellington at the Battle of Waterloo and he got his leg shot off and he's reported to have said, "Damn, I've had my leg shot off!"[5] That expresses the phlegmatic temperament, yeah?

---

[4] Vasant Lad, *Ayurveda—the Science of Self-Healing: A Practical Guide* (Lotus Press, 1993). [Ed.]

[5] Christopher is referring to Henry Paget, the cavalry commander at the Battle of Waterloo. The Duke of Wellington is said to have replied to Paget's outcry at the loss of his leg by saying, "By God, sir, so you have!", also reflecting more than a degree of "phlegmatocity", a term that Christopher liked to use. You may or may not like to know that after his victory, the Duke asked his shoemaker to design a new boot, using soft calfskin to the knee. As a war hero, the new boot caught on, and is the origin of the Wellington boot, or "Wellies", even if now they have a reduced height and are made of rubber or pvc and are generally not regarded as the height of fashion by most people, except at Glastonbury, of course. Christopher preferred good walking boots. [Ed.]

Beware of angry phlegmatics

Phlegmatic people do feel. Phlegmatic people are watery. They're like the ocean. They feel and they feel very deeply, but they don't let you know. Again, they're like the ocean, I'd rather have any other humour angry with me than a phlegmatic person, because by the time they get round to expressing their anger to me, I'm dead! Keep in with your phlegmatic friends. Bear in mind that it's all going on down there at a deep level. So, phlegmatic people are watery people. There's a physical shape, of course. This is not just an emotional system; this is a physical system as well. The nice thing about any constitutional medicine is that we are integrating the whole person, the physical person, the emotional person, everything goes together. So, it is basically, absolutely and unalterably, a holistic way of looking at things. The physical shape of phlegmatic people is pear-shaped, because water sinks. So, therefore, phlegmatic people tend to be pale skinned and pear shaped. I always think of the, you know the expression the "English Rose"? Very pale skin, I always think of a pear-shaped English rose, when I think of phlegmatic people.

Water sinks

Which is the phlegmatic person in Winnie the Pooh? This is really hard because phlegmatic people hide. It's Piglet, Piglet is the phlegmatic person in Winnie the Pooh! And you can actually tell from the pictures because he is that shape, yeah, he's pear-shaped, basically, Piglet. If you look at those little pictures, the last one in the book of him and Pooh going away, with a very classic pear shape. Of course, water sinks, so phlegmatic people tend to be pear-shaped.

Two big things

Water does two big things. It flows, so it encourages flowing and movement, so it's lubrication. It also binds, sticks together, as in making sandcastles. You cannot make a sandcastle out of dry sand; you need the water to stick together. So, water binds. So, those are the main two characteristics of watery people—flowingness and bindingness.

Phlegmatocity

So, phlegmatic people, they're heavy, they tend to drag, they tend to be really soft and slow, their features are round, fairly indistinct, squashy noses, something like that. Their skin is cool and pale. They will not meet your gaze, they'll tend to look away. There will be wateriness about their eyes. You cannot be aggressive with a watery person. You can't be in their face, it's quite difficult, you have to be directive but not pushy. The pulse will usually be quite hidden, you have to really feel for it. The circulation will be cold. They'll feel the cold easily. Probably the most important pathological thing is because they're cold and damp, they have no digestive heat, so they suffer a lot from indigestion, candidiasis, whatever that is, that sort of thing with a mucousy-looking tongue. Tongue's always mucousy-looking. They tend to bloating, with mucus in the stools, irritable bowel type thing. So, one of the most important things with phlegmatic people is to get them to eat warm food, not raw food, but warm food and use gentle spices not harsh spices. The interesting thing about that, of course, is that the classical, traditional English diet was quite spicy. If you read Mrs Beeton[6], for example, she was chucking in spices right, left and centre, which is more suitable for balancing the excess phlegmatocity of English people.

Be friendly and move on

One of the interesting things that Culpeper says about herbs is that you give a herb that appropriates to the humour and then we give other herbs that pull the humour round to where you want it to be, if you see what I mean? It's no good just saying, this person is very cold and dry, let's fill them up with hot water. It won't work. You need to give something which addresses the earth. Actually, the best example of that is giving medicines based on milk to phlegmatic people with coughs. It's logical, it's a logical thing to do because if the phlegm is stuck, if you give milk it will promote more flow of phlegm and therefore unstick the thick phlegm, yes? It's the logical thing to do. But I tend to give

---

[6] Isabella Mary Beeton (1836–1865), known as Mrs Beeton, was an English writer. She is particularly well known for her first book, the 1861 work *Mrs Beeton's Book of Household Management*, which is still in print. See: Isabella Beeton, *Mrs. Beeton's Book of Household Management: The 1861 Classic with Advice on Cooking, Cleaning, Childrearing, Entertaining, and More.* (Western Classics, 2020). [Ed.]

my grandfather's favourite remedy which was milk and Cinnamon and brandy and I think this is what happens—the milk comes up to the phlegm and the phlegm says, "Well, you look like a nice person to hang around with, I recognise something in you, I'll hang around with you." And then in goes the brandy and Cinnamon and does the job. I love that. So that balances out promoting the humour but also moving it on. Being friendly with the humour but also moving it on. It's extremely important.

It's a job to remember

Phlegm hides emotions, phlegm reflects. Water reflects, it reflects on past events. When you get older the phlegm becomes dominant and old memories become clear, the deep stuff at the bottom of the pool starts to come up and becomes clear and you lose, you forget where you've put the keys and whatever, but that's OK, that's allowed, that's how it should be because the job of old people is to remember. The job of elders is to remember, that's what they do. And they remember their life not just for themselves but for everybody. So, you let them remember. It's very, very important because then that provides continuity. One of the darn things that's wrong with this society is we don't honour old people, so we don't allow them to remember. We just bombard them with adverts saying you can still be climbing Mount Everest when you're ninety-four, which is OK, I mean if you want to, but we don't allow them to remember. So, we lose our continuity. And in traditional societies, of course, old people would remember, and the young children were always put in the care of the old people in order to be taught the old ways and to provide the continuity. And that doesn't happen.

Hydraulic engines

Probably the best word to use about phlegmatic people is lethargy. Lethargic is not the same as depressed, it means heavy. It means your body feels heavy, just sat there. Like you feel Christmas evening watching, I like to watch "The Wizard of Oz" myself, don't you? As you're sat there on your couch, getting more and more lethargic. They dislike exercise, it's quite difficult to get them to exercise. They tend to be passive, they tend to be covetous, stingy and conservative, careful and dependable. As I said, they feel their emotions deeply but they will hide them. On the good side they are kind and friendly, and they're very practical. They are very, very stubborn, which is a power to be reckoned with. You don't make hydraulic engines out of fire, you make them out of water, yeah?

The Melancholy Humour

Melilot haze

Culpeper, of course, was famously a choleric melancholic. Fire and earth. He wrote something like forty books and translated other books, most of which have gone, and he died at thirty-five or something. But, he was prone to episodes of melancholy and getting stuck and not doing anything. So, his herbal is full of remedies for melancholy. So, one of his favourite remedies for melancholy was baths in Lemon Balm. Another thing is baths in Melilot. Melilot's nice. If you want to get rid of melancholic feelings in the house, hang Melilot up, because the smell goes on for ages and ages, which is down to its coumarin chemistry. So, the smell goes on for ages and ages and it gives you this nice, light, clear haze, yes, nice and light and clear. So, I do that every year. Hang up a nice bunch of Melilot in the house.

Out to the heavens

Melancholic people—you need herbs which are moving and cleansing and gently warming but not too warm, because there's no point in setting fire to the earth. It'd be like those coal mines that just burn and burn for thirty or forty years, that's no good. But gentle warming things like Angelica and Fennel. Mostly umbelliferous herbs actually, which is interesting isn't it? Because they're all up and out to the sky and out to the heavens, they balance the heaviness like that.

What do you expect, really

Melancholics are very careful, can be fearful and even tight fisted. General air of being worn out. Suffer in silence. Who is the melancholy character in Winne the Pooh? The quote from Eeyore was, "I'm not complaining, but there it is." And of course, when Eeyore built a house, Winnie the Pooh mistook it for a pile of sticks. Because they're not really that interested in material purities and things like that. I love the bit where he's floating down the river. It's just, "What do you expect, really." And then they try to rescue him by throwing rocks at him.

Permission granted

They tend to be antisocial. Tend to like their own company. The difference between melancholia and depression is that melancholic people like being melancholic. I did have someone come to me after a workshop and say, "You've just saved my marriage!" Her husband was very melancholic, and he'd often go and sit in his room all by himself and she'd come and try and cheer him up. "I used to worry about it but I shan't worry about it anymore." It worked really well. As a melancholic, you need time by yourself. It's very difficult in this society. You must realise that people with any strong earthy element must have time to themselves just to be, just to be. The key word for fire is doing and the key word for earth is being. Just be. So, basically, often with patients, just give them permission to be who they are.

You can upset an earthy person

They're introverted, obviously. A tendency to sadness or pessimism. Stubborn. Obstinate. Suspicious. They retain anger. You can, if you wish, upset an earthy person because they will remember but they don't necessarily do anything about it. The organ in which earth is said most to reside is the spleen because the spleen in traditional medicine is the organ that makes you physically, the physical you. It's to do with digestion and absorption. And the spleen likes to be a little bit dry and a little bit cold. It doesn't like to be wet at all. So, that term "splenic" applies very well to an earthy person's anger. They'll just hold on to it and hold on to it and hold on to it. And then maybe they'll come out and get you, but they would probably just beat themselves up really.

Unsticking an astrologer

I had a client with a melancholic disposition. I had a long and interesting conversation with him because he's an astrologer. I don't really know much astrology but I know the terminology so I can have long conversations with him. He got really, really stuck. He was writing a book and, being of a melancholic disposition, it was taking him a very, very, very, very long time and he was crafting each letter, practically, in the book. Making sure that everything said precisely and exactly what he wanted. And it was taking him so long that his ideas where actually developing while he was writing the book. Then he was having to go back and rewrite and he was just getting nowhere at all. And he got total, complete writer's block. And the simplest solution was just to put Clary Sage essential oil in an oil burner. Sit down, light the oil burner before you write. It worked really well. It's very light, moving, uplifting, took away that heaviness from him. I can't understand a word, well I can understand words in the book, I just can't understand the book actually, to tell you the truth. He gave me a copy, I'm sure it's a very nice book. It's so dense. Wow!

Like rocks

Their skin tends to be dark or ashen. Often itchy because they're dry. Their eyes would be dark and usually dull, and they'd avoid eye contact. They tend to have a lack of bodily hair. Their pulse would be heavy, unsteady and slow. They tend to overheat in hot weather, like rocks.

New ways

I'd just like to share something the American herbalist jim mcdonald found on a website for a Swedish raincoat manufacturer[7] about melancholy, people of an earthy constitution, popular in Sweden I understand. Melancholy is the most misunderstood constitution in our society and, because melancholy's about being, earth is about being and this society's all about doing isn't it? Why do we have to have economic growth for God's sake, why can't we just live? I don't know. Anyway, this is the quote, "Melancholy shouldn't be confused with depression. Melancholy is an active state. When we're melancholic, we feel uneasy with the way things are, the status quo, the conventions of our society. We yearn for a deeper, richer relationship with the world. And in that yearning, we're forced to explore the potential within ourselves—a potential we might not have explored if we were simply content. Through our melancholy we come up with new ways

---

[7] If you fancy a raincoat with this story attached to it, the company is Stutterheim. [Ed.]

of seeing the world and new ways of being in the world. Melancholy and creativity go together like ebony and ivory on a piano." Buy my mackintosh! Lovely, isn't it?

Let's face it

Earthy people are cold and dry. They tend to be of fairly slight build, but the way to spot them is by sallowness of the complexion. So, there's a slight grey sheen to their skin. They're very stubborn. Earthy people are the exact opposite of fiery people, in that they will hang in there, and if you want to treat an earthy person, a melancholic person, then what you've got to say is, "Well, getting better is a big job, let's face it. It's really hard and it's going to take you all your life."

Walk four hundred miles

You say, "OK, melancholic person, why don't you go out and play squash." They look at you as if you were mad, of course, yes? If you say to the melancholic person, "Why don't you take up long distance walking? There are some really nice trails, two three, four hundred miles long now, you can go up the mountains." Invariably what they'd say is, "I used to do that when I was young." Because we do know, we actually do know what's right for us, because sometime in our life we've done it and we felt that it's right for us. So, long country walks. If they haven't got time to do that, they can walk into work, that sort of thing.

Dual-function thistles for Eeyore

Melancholy tends to build up in the liver and melancholic people are particularly prone to liver congestion. The melancholic person in Winnie the Pooh is, of course, Eeyore. And what did Eeyore eat? Eeyore ate Thistles. Now partially, no doubt, he ate Thistles because he could say, "I'm having to eat all this horrible, prickly stuff." But actually, Thistles are the best liver herbs, among the best liver herbs. All Thistles are good liver herbs. So, he wasn't so daft, he was stopping the congestion building up in his liver. Artichokes are Thistles, yes, my favourite liver decongestive is Artichokes with Garlic and butter sauce, olive oil if I'm feeling good, you can practically feel your liver going, "Thank you, thank you!"

The Humours Together

Is

Fire is doing, isn't it? Doing is highly valued in this society, particularly for men. "I know, let's go and chop that forest down." It must be good, because we're doing something.

Water is feeling and emotions. If you've got a watery person in front of you, you can talk in terms of feelings. You can say, "How do you feel about this?" So, feeling is underrated in this society, but probably always was. The phlegmatic person feels things, but they don't tell you that they're feeling things. They're not going to talk about it, they're going to just feel it.

Air is thinking. Airy people like to think. They love new ideas. Journalists are the classic airy people. I have a friend who's a journalist. When she's writing an article on something she knows everything there is to know about it and if you ask her the week after and she's forgotten. Quite amazing. Never ceases to amaze me. Earth is being, and that is the most underrated thing in this society. Just being. Just sitting being is the most underrated thing, and it's the thing that we really need the most of. We need to identify melancholic people and immediately make them all senators, don't we?

Express yourself

When you find you have two dominant humours, the most important thing is to allow expression. So, for example, if you have fire and water, use the fieriness in your work and the wateriness at home. So, be really fiery at work and then be really watery at home. Work's a suitable environment, of course, to be fiery, push, push, push and go for it, and then you get home and can be all emotional and soft and soggy in there, with children around you, and so on and so forth. That's a very good way to do it.

Shape shifting

I had a patient a few years ago, she was fire and water, she still is fire and water, isn't she? And she'd got totally stuck in wateriness, because she was married to a guy who was English and a bit anally retentive type and hiding his stuff and a lot of people want to share their emotions.

And she was teaching in a school, which is going to bring out your wateriness basically, you know, softness and so on. And she was extremely large and at her most watery she actually started oozing phlegm out of her tummy button. I've never seen anything quite like it. She was full of phlegm—wateriness and wateriness, and it was very interesting because she was a Tibetan Buddhist, well she wasn't Tibetan, but you know what I mean. She went away and did a three-month retreat, she worked her way up to a three-month retreat, and decided to change her whole life around. She came back, she left her partner, said I don't want any divorce settlement, I'm just going to go. She moved across to Holland and found a nice young man and got a job as an organiser of meditation centres, and when I saw her, like she came knocking on my door saying, "I haven't seen you for a bit", her whole shape had changed. It was amazing. It was like seeing a different person. She was all fiery, and of course what happened then is she started to suffer from fiery things. So, then you have to balance them both.

Comfort and calm

Usually, of course, when you see patients, most people have fallen ill because they let one humour get over the top. So, it's much easier to see the patterns in patients than it is in ourselves, because something is dominating, quite clearly something is dominating, and then you deal with that, but then you do not neglect the other things. So, a friend of mine is very sanguine, but he's got quite a lot of wateriness, so I recommended for him, always put a bit of Mallow or something nice and soft, it's a very simple medicine but it works. So, comfort the humours. Comfort the humours that need comforting and calm down the humours that need calming down, basically.

Being run over by a truck

One of my favourite teaching things to sort of pin it down, is to think what happens if you get run over by a truck. What does a choleric person do if they're run over by a truck? They get angry. They get up and they kick the truck and break their leg, don't they? Yes. What does a phlegmatic person do when run over by a truck? They cry, but they'd probably go away and do it where no one can see. They'll get up and they'll walk away and they'll go round behind a tree and have a little cry.

What does a sanguine person do when run over by a truck? They jump up and scream and then something new happens and they'll forget all about it. What does a melancholic person do when run over by a truck? They'd just lie there and say, "Yes, what do you expect, why don't you do it again?"

A United Nations decree

So, the quality of the land tends to bring out those aspects within people and people will go and live there. It's very interesting, I notice this in America because people can easily move between different climate zones, you can't really do that in Europe. People tend to accumulate in places that, it's ever so interesting, that suit their humours. I sometimes think that the best thing the United Nations could do was just give grants to people to move to wherever they wanted to, and everybody would be happy and there wouldn't be any war, would there? And you wouldn't all finish up in the South of France, people like different places, or California. People like different places, absolutely.

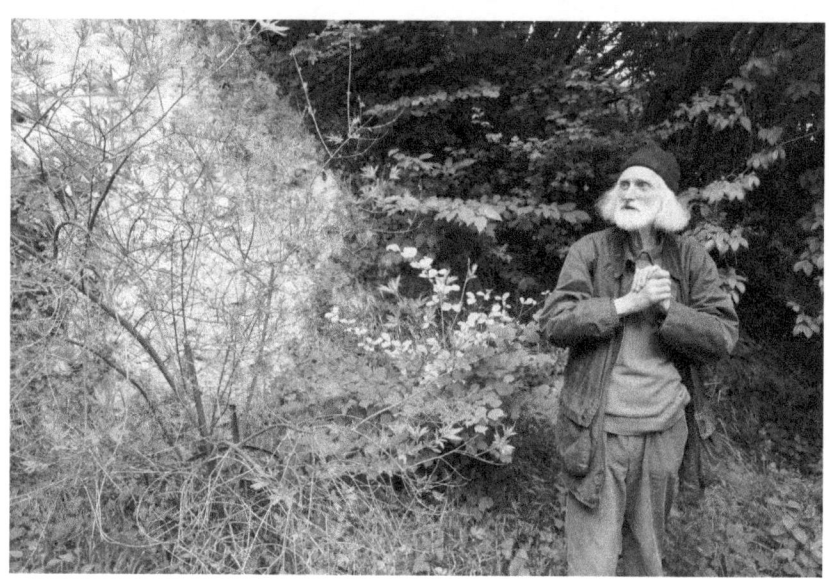

Photo by Bruno Pires

Flowers—Materia Medica of Plant Medicine

Artist's Bracket (*Ganoderma applanatum*)

Must be soupy

I always use fungus extracts as a simple, alongside any other medicine I may give, as it's the only way to get a reasonable dose. It means lots of time spent in making, but that after all is only fun. I haven't found fresh plant extracts to be better than dried so I prefer freshly dried, although I keep some in case I run out of extract before the season starts.

I use mainly Artist's Bracket (*G. applanatum*), which is dirt common around here. I have found the fungus growing on Birch to be best. I originally selected it because it is smaller and denser than that growing on larger trees, and it is more bitter. Reishi (*G. lucidum*) is very rare here so not practical. I also use Lacquered Bracket (*G. resinaceum*) which is quite rare but which grows freely in my local park—kind of it! This is always quite sweet and I use it when the patient needs sweetness.

We also have here, in the UK, Shelf Fungus (*G. adspersum*), which is more common, thicker and even more perennial than the *G. applanatum*. I am of the opinion that the thinner species make the best medicines. They have a more resinous coat and a larger tube layer per unit volume and thus, perhaps, a wider variety of constituents in the final extract. I feel that the resinous coat is an important part of the fungi. I have used other methods but I tend to agree that making a tincture first and then a decoction of the same material gives the best results. I have used this preparation for some three years now. I am convinced of its use for anxiety associated with serious disease and I have one case of hepatitis C with significant cirrhosis who only responded after I added the Ganoderma to her original mixture—taken as a decoction since we were worried about any alcohol. I use it consistently in HIV but have yet to find it of value in cancer.

It seems to me that the methods described that use 50% alcohol and then combine it with the reduced decoction gets the best of both worlds, phytochemically speaking. But, I am most interested in the polysaccharides, so I go for a final strength of 20% alcohol. I don't know why everyone uses 25%. It seems to me the lower the alcohol the better, given the notorious instability of big, jolly polysaccharides. I also add 10% glycerine and vitamin C, which is said to improve absorption and should improve preservation. However, you do it, the final extract must be soupy. It is this quality that makes for really deep level immune system nourishing. I am happy to have the bitter triterpenes but I don't feel them getting as deep into the system as the polysaccharides. It is very important when treating immune system dysfunction to use herbs that get below the level of the damage.[1]

Host to host

I have never seen mentioned the possibility of differences in the fungi due to different hosts, although there are differences in taste. I have noticed that the softer bracket fungi taste quite different from host to host. The Sulphur Polypore (*Laetiporus sulphureus*) is quite tasty when growing on Oak or Willow but is disturbingly Yew-tasting when growing on Yew—so much so that I couldn't bring myself to eat it. *G. applanatum* grows mostly on Beech (*Fagus sylvatica*) here and I have mostly used it from Beech; it is generally sweet and a little bitter.

---

[1] Please see Seeds, "Get below", this volume. [Ed.]

Astragalus (Astragalus mongholicus syn. A. membranaceus)
Approaching sideways with a story

I was pondering on Astragalus for another way of looking at it. The herb is basically a strengthener of the spleen. As understood in traditional medicine, the spleen makes your earth, your substance. Astragalus is a pea and pea roots strengthen the ground in which they grow. The spleen holds things, good and bad. That is what it does. It might hold the bug as well but that is OK if you add in a bug-killer since the spleen's holding makes the job of Woad (*Isatis tinctoria*) even easier. Just a story, but stories are what count. There is no way of describing the actual truth of things so we have to approach it sideways with stories.

Balm, Lemon Balm (*Melissa officinalis*)
We didn't have nerves

Lemon Balm is a cordial. In the old words that means it's a heart medicine. "Coeur", French word. That's the heart, isn't it? Sure, it is. Cordial is a heart medicine. If you drink Lemon Balm tea you can try this yourself at home, it's perfectly safe. Drink some Lemon Balm tea and look for what we call the appropriations of the herb. Where the herb likes to go to in the body. Different herbs have different appropriations, they have different parts of the body they go to. Some herbs are quite dispersant and go to many parts. Lemon Balm is a herb that goes straight to the heart centre and you can feel it there straightaway. You can feel it even more definitely than Hawthorn. Straight into the heart centre, clears and calms the heart centre. Uplifts the spirit, gets the vital spirits going from where they're residing in the heart. So, nowadays we'd call that a nervine, in the old days, of course, we didn't have nerves. Nerves are a new invention and they'd say, "It's a heart remedy." That's nicer, isn't it? I think we could do without nerves, don't you? Nowadays, we call it a nervine. In William Salmon's *Pharmacopoeia Londinensis*[2] of 1696, Lemon Balm "comforts the Stomach, removes Melancholy, cheers the Heart, causes pleasant Dreams, expels Poyson, cures the Plague", and an

---

[2] William Salmon, *Pharmacopoeia Londinensis, Or, the New London Dispensatory* (T. Baffett, R. Chifwell, M. Wotton, G. Conyers and I. Dawks, 1696), 76–77. https://archive.org/details/bim_early-english-books-1641-1700_pharmacopoeia-londinensi_salmon-william_1696/page/28/mode/2up. [Ed.]

essence made of Lemon Balm, Greater Celandine, Poppy flowers and Rosemary "renews Youth, keeps back old Age ... strengthens the Brain, restores lost Memory, relieves languishing Nature ... and prevents Gray Hairs and Baldness..." Pretty good?

Bittersweet (Solanum dulcamara)

Six inches

The only thing I have used it for is in helping men maintain an erection. It does work. Simply chew a six inch piece of fresh twig. Many Solanaceae have the same action. I use a low alcohol tincture of the fresh two- to three-year-old stems, picked in the autumn. I have tried it for psoriasis, without success—but I think I chose the wrong people.

Rudolph Weiss[3] makes the point that Solanums *per se* have atropine-like properties to a greater or lesser extent. He has an interesting story concerning a patient who was taking potato water for gastritis and who developed blurred vision which cleared up when the potato water was stopped. So, possibly part of its activity in skin disease is the anticholinergic effect—pulling blood away from the peripheral circulation. The herb also has an alterative action. Weiss recommends it for arthritis and chronic skin disease. Other sources recommend it for chronic catarrh and asthma, which may also be down to an anticholinergic action similar to Datura.

It had a use in folk medicine for cancer but has fallen from favour. Julian Barker[4] makes the point that this may be because there are several chemotypes. Reading all I can find and trying it for myself I am of the opinion that Bittersweet will work best on phlegmatic people and phlegm blockage and thus probably most useful for elders. Anyway, I am motivated to try again this autumn.

Boneset (Eupatorium perfoliatum)

Poured it down his throat

Fiery people can get very high temperatures, so herbs which reduce high temperatures and break high fevers are useful herbs to have around if you've got fiery people in the house. I'm reminded of my friend, who's actually

---

[3] Rudolf Fritz Weiss, *Herbal Medicine* (Arcanum, 1988). [Ed].

[4] Julian Barker, *The Medicinal Flora of Britain & Northwest Europe: A Field Guide, Including Plants Commonly Cultivated in the Region* (West Wickham, Kent: Winter Press, 2001). [Ed.]

a herbalist, who is a very fiery person, bright red hair, bounces around, and he got ill. He got ill in a way that fiery people get ill, he just totally ignored his body and went on working. Actually, it's the way that herbalists and I'm sure naturopaths, get ill as well, isn't it? You've just got people to treat, haven't you? You've got to ignore yourself. So, he ignored himself, he ignored himself and it got up to Christmas, stopped work, crash, out on the floor, temperature of 200 degrees or something, delirious. His wife says he was lying on the floor delirious. Never seen anybody delirious before. Really frightening. Won't take any medicine. "No, I'm all right, I don't want any medicine, go away." So, after a while, after about a few hours of not getting any reaction, she went and got some Boneset and she boiled up the Boneset, a really, really thick treacly decoction of about two kilos of Boneset in it and held his nose and poured it down his throat and his fever broke and he was all right, and that's basically how you treat fiery people. Short term goals I think is an important one. Give them something they can go for within the short term. It is a waste of time talking about health as a long-term thing. Just do it short term.[5]

Borage (*Borago officinalis*)

How happy they are

An ex-student did her MSc research on the pyrrolizidine alkaloid content of Borage. She tested the total pyrrolizidine alkaloid content of plants and tinctures from a variety of sources. She found very high levels in tincture produced by a large (very commercial) firm who imported their Borage and almost zero levels in plants grown for her by a small producer. She told me that those plants were very obviously happy plants. The small producer has a walled garden and grows her herbs scattered throughout it and mixed together. Larger commercial firms will grow herbs in monocultures. Pyrrolizidine alkaloids are antifeedants and insects are less attracted to mixed gardens and more to monocultures—so that is one explanation, but I prefer this one—happy plants are healthy plants and make good medicine. So, talk to your plants, tell them why you are picking them and ask them how happy they are.[6]

---

[5] As Boneset contains pyrrolizidine alkaloids, please keep up to date on the research and debates around hepatotoxicity of medicinal plants that contain this constituent. [Ed.]

[6] Similarly to Boneset, above, please keep up to date on the research and debates about pyrrolizidine alkaloids and hepatotoxicity. [Ed.]

Cayenne (*Capsicum annuum* syn. *C. frutescens*)
He was red

My favourite story about Cayenne concerns the beginner's class that I teach, it's two hours once a week over the winter. A few years ago, I was teaching a class and there was a man who came in, he sat at the back of the class and he was the colour of concrete and, I kind of, I expected him to die. Anyway, he came for three or four weeks and then he stopped coming and I thought, "Oh he's died!" Next year he turned up again at the beginning of class and he was a totally different colour, he was red, there was a spring in his step, he was a healthy person. So, I got him down the café quickly and I said, "Tell me how you did this!" We had a cup of tea, he gets a little dropper bottle out of his pocket and it contained Cayenne tincture. And he said, "All I do is I put four or five drops of Cayenne tincture in every single drink I drink, that's all I've done for the year." It was quite amazing. It's a really powerful technique.

Chaste Berry (*Vitex agnus-castus*)
Monk's pepper grinder

Vitex will normalise high or low testosterone levels so it is useful for monks with a high sex drive. One method was to put it into a pepper grinder and use it as a condiment. In that case all the monks ate it. Female libido is much more complex than that of men and I have heard of women who took Vitex at the menopause, whose libido increased.

A funny feeling

OK, so there is something of a debate over here on Vitex doses. The general tendency is to use say 20 drops of a 1:5 once daily, first thing in the morning for PMS, for example[7]. I'm not quite sure where the first thing in the morning came from but it works (Madaus Pharma used to recommend that strategy). I usually express it as, "Hit the pituitary whilst it is still working out what settings to use that day." A total daily dose of 3 ml

---

[7] This was written a while ago now, and the general UK herbal practice of Vitex dosing for PMS (still often given in the morning) seems to have increased a bit, to about 10 drops of a fluid extract (1:1), which is theoretically about 2.5 times the dose Christopher mentioned. Of course, it is difficult to standardise herbalists or herbal practice. As Christopher used to say, if you put people in boxes, their arms and legs stick out. [Ed.]

is more the level of dose for pituitary tumours, or for men wishing to lower their sex drive, or for women wishing to raise their libido.

But, perhaps dosage should not be an issue. I have a funny feeling that once I start thinking too much about that then the herb slips and slides into a drug. That is, I might think of it as suppressing physiology (oestrogen dependence, testosterone, etc.) rather than as supporting and encouraging it. I should be thinking more about when, and for what type of person, to use it. My teacher used to say, for example, "Take care when using Vitex with people prone to headaches and with severe, congestive menstrual pain." The herb warns me, for example, it is too easy to use it to start up menstruation when stopped, but things won't hold unless I think of the whole picture as well.

Herbs change lives

I have a friend who uses only the leaves on the grounds that they work just as well and the yield is better. After all, most people in the world use the leaves of most species of Vitex most of the time.

A couple of stories from patients. One lady who thought that her Vitex drops were the best thing I gave her—and I gave her several things to take, as it is a favourite strategy of mine to split the herbs into separate medicines, so that people can hear what the herbs have to say to their bodies and respond separately to them. She said that the drops helped her to get started in the morning—it does have a good, tingly taste. I have had other patients who used Vitex for mild depression/lethargy. I wonder if this corelates to its use for obsessions? Another lady who was given Vitex for severe premenstrual depression, amongst many other things, reported a few months later that her whole life was in better balance—the words were her own. Herbs change lives.

Comfrey (Symphytum officinale)

People and cats

The best and most clear statement on the activity of Comfrey is by Simon Mills in his "Essential Book of Herbal Medicine", which is, by the way and in my opinion, by far the best book he has written. I quote, "Allantoin ... promotes the constructive activity of the fibroblasts in producing connective tissue, and their near relatives the chondroblasts (cartilage) and osteoblasts (bone) and even neural cells, it promotes keratin dispersal ... it thus aids the regeneration of all tissues ... with the possible exception of skeletal muscle ... In addition, allantoin is highly diffusible through the body and can be relied upon to reach deep tissues from external application."[8]

In some cases, the keratinolytic action of Comfrey predominates. People and cats with thin skin have to be careful and not use it for too long, on the other hand it makes a good application for corns. I always use it as my base for bone spur creams and for keloid scars and such.

Culpeper[9] says that Comfrey is useful for gout and joint pains. In those days the most common type of arthritis must have been osteoarthritis, which involves bone growing unevenly, too much in one place, too little in another. Interestingly, Culpeper seems to be describing Tuberous Comfrey (*S. tuberosum*) as the most important. It may well have been the common Comfrey in Spitalfields, which was a market garden area in his time. Tuberous Comfrey has the lowest pyrrolizidine alkaloid content in the genus.[10]

Nibbling up

Something very interesting about maggots—basically allantoin. Have you heard of allantoin, from Comfrey? Amazing. So, not only do they go around nibbling up necrotic tissue, they're secreting allantoin, which makes the good tissue grow.[11] Where did that come from? I don't know, sometimes I think it's all a plot, don't you?

---

[8] Simon Mills, *The Essential Book of Herbal Medicine* (Penguin, 1993), 545. [Ed.]

[9] Culpeper, *Culpeper's Complete Herbal*, 76–77. Please see footnote 10, below, highlighting safety concerns of Comfrey.

[10] Similarly to Boneset and Borage, above, please keep an eye on the research and debates around pyrrolizidine alkaloid hepatoxicity. Comfrey root is not currently recommended for internal use in the UK, and some authorities and professional associations also caution against any internal use of the leaf, which has lower levels of this constituent, while others allow its use for short periods only. [Ed.]

[11] Please see the following two sources, the first of which is a wide-ranging review of larvae that are parasitic on vertebrates, which includes confirmation of allantoin production, while the second source investigates the mechanism of production of allantoin through purine catabolism in medical maggots.
Philip Scholl, Douglas Colwell, and Ramón Cepeda-Palacios, "Myiasis (Muscoidea, Oestrodea)," in *Medical and Veterinary Entomology*, ed. Gary Mullen and Lance Durden (Elsevier Inc., 2019), 384–419.
Andre Baumann et al., "Urate Oxidase Produced by Lucilia Sericata Medical Maggots Is Localized in Malpighian Tubes and Facilitates Allantoin Production," *Insect Biochemistry and Molecular Biology* 83 (April 1, 2017): 44–53, https://doi.org/10.1016/j.ibmb.2017.02.007. [Ed.]

Cramp Bark (*Viburnum opulus*)

Go by the smell

One thing about the Viburnums, we have two species here; *Viburnum opulus* and *Viburnum lantana* and only the *opulus* works as a good herb for relaxing spasm. I suspect that only some Viburnum species are useful—it's easy to tell, go by the smell, looking for that distinctive salicylate aroma. I wouldn't like to use the root bark, as it involves digging the tree up, when the stem bark works well and it coppices easily. I always use it with a little Ginger—for added zoom.

Echinacea, Coneflower (*Echinacea* spp.)

Even on herbalists themselves

One problem with Coneflower is that when taking for long periods people do not back it up with herbs that offer support to the rest of the system. Again, this is a mistake made with other herbs as well but arises more often with herbs that are used by non-herbally aware sections of the population, especially the trendy extensively "researched" herbs. Such attitudes tend to rub off, even on herbalists themselves. It is difficult to resist the all-pervading intent of society, hence the need to constantly reacquaint ourselves with the herbs themselves. They at least are immune to human follies.

I used to keep an infused oil of Golden Seal and Ground Ivy for use in tinnitus and found it very helpful. Also, I tend to use Ground Ivy with Echinacea for colds and flu. I find that one part of Echinacea to two parts of Ground Ivy works better than the equivalent amount of Echinacea alone, thus enabling me to use less Echinacea. Perhaps next year I will use Ground Ivy and Elderberries and keep the Echinacea for the serious stuff it is best at.

For people with good vitality suffering from recurrent infections following immune system stress I will use Echinacea in smaller doses for longer periods BUT only in combination with "deeper" acting, more supportive, herbs. The classic example is recurrent minor infection in children following prolonged antibiotic use. My typical protocol is Siberian Ginseng and Echinacea, equal parts, take 5 ml, two or three times daily for two or three months.

Of interest, try Echinacea as a simple for early infections with swollen lymph nodes. Echinacea will often reduce the swelling but it quickly comes back. Adding Poke root will bring the swelling down and keep it down.

Pushy regimes

Orthodox treatments, especially steroids, of course, weaken the body's vital reserves and might be expected to precipitate a bad reaction to Echinacea. It is very noticeable that patients who have never been on steroids respond more quickly and more pushy regimes can be used. Diminished vitality allows diseases to get under the immune system's immediate defenses. For example, influenza going to the blood level with recurrent fever and deep aches. Classic sweating herbs such as Elderflower and Yarrow are more useful here than Echinacea.

Need a good vitality to work with

These days I use only *Echinacea purpurea* (fresh plant tincture 1:2)—mainly because of ecological issues. One of my suppliers makes a combined root and green seed fresh plant tincture which is a very nice preparation—but then she makes very good medicines in general. I keep her whole plant specific tincture for use with children and sensitive individuals.

In common with many herbalists, I prefer to use Echinacea in high doses for short periods, e.g. in bringing a tooth abscess under control when I typically use 20 drops every two hours. The key point being frequent doses for a short period. I have also brought septicaemia under control with 5 ml every two hours. I have seen this several times when helping with first aid at festivals—in basically healthy individuals with septicaemia following deep wounds.

People do not take enough when dealing with acute symptoms. This mistake is made with other herbs as well and is often due, in Europe anyway, to the inflated price of over-the-counter preparations. A brief look at the dosage levels in the Eclectic literature[12] should break this habit.

---

[12] Key authors in the Eclectic tradition include John Uri Lloyd, Harvey Wickes Felter, Finlay Ellingwood, John M Scudder, and Eli Jones. Please see Henriette Kress's awesome website for a treasure trove of historical resources, including Eclectic texts: www.henriettes-herb.com [Ed.]

E. pallida seems to work as a dried herb whereas *E. purpurea* does not. For adults with deeper damage to the immune system but with still enough vitality to suffer from "ordinary" symptoms of recurrent, minor infections I often add a little *Echinacea pallida* to a long-term decoction of more deeper acting herbs. For example, hepatitis C with not too much obvious damage. The key factor being the strength of the vital spirit. Echinacea needs a good vitality to work with. The more diminished the vital response the less useful is Echinacea.

Disordered or loose heat

It seems to me that treatment of autoimmune patients with Echinacea depends on the activity of the condition. These diseases can burn themselves out. This is most obvious in late rheumatoid arthritis when symptoms are mainly due to joint damage and active inflammation is low. In such cases, Echinacea may be used to treat infections in the same way as in "healthy" people. I have followed this course many times with no adverse reactions.

My dosing is of the order of 10 to 15 ml a day but for short periods only, usually 10 days. If the infection is not brought under control in this time, then other strategies are needed. If the disease is still very active then Echinacea does not work. This is most obvious in connective tissue diseases such as SLE, sarcoidosis etc., when the patient is still showing signs of loose fire. In such cases, Echinacea is not useful and the classic cooling strategies, such as demonstrated by *Eupatorium* spp. Are more helpful: the vital spirit has been undermined and the vital response is low, manifesting as disordered or loose heat, and the Echinacea has nothing to work with. I can see that, in such cases, Echinacea might even be counterproductive.

Elecampane (Inula helenium)

Chunky

A very striking and robust plant, as broad as it is high, chunky is a good word for it, prefers deeper moisture from retentive soil in partial shade, likes woodland edges. Elecampane says to me, "I am a strong and sunny plant with a strong root and sunny flowers, use me to strengthen and bulk up weak people." And indeed, the first use of Elecampane is to strengthen digestion for people who are wasting or people who have lost their appetite. Elecampane root in this sense is a true spleen herb, using spleen in the proper sense of the word which is the organ that makes you out of the food you eat. The spleen of course is the seat of melancholy in traditional medicine, and the particular type of anger that comes from accumulations of melancholy venting the spleen.

A big hacking cough

Inula helenium is supposed to be named after Helen of Troy, which makes my think that Helen of Troy may or may not have been beautiful but she definitely had a nasty cough. I think, my own personal theory is that Paris is walking around the countryside and hears this big hacking cough from the other side of the hedge, and he comes round the corner, there's Helen, "Hack! Hack! Hack!" And Paris, like lots of traditional families, had a recipe passed down by his granny, in traditional societies a lot of families have two or three recipes which they pass down, and he was very, very proud of the cough medicine he'd got from his granny. So, he gave it to Helen, and she got better, and he immediately fell in love and started the whole wooden horse thing. I think of Elecampane as a lung restorative. A restorative is a herb which is applicable to any condition of that particular organ, it restores any condition whatsoever.

All lung diseases

I think Elecampane is applicable to all lung disease, even asthma, you need to take it for a while though, and the decoction is best because you get the soothing as well as the slightly sharp edge out of it. The only possible drawback is pointed out by William Cook[13], lovely writing. It tends to be dry and tends to be too dry for dry lung conditions, but that's easy dealt with, isn't it? Just by adding something nice and soft like Coltsfoot or Mallow or Comfrey, I do like Comfrey[14]. I like

---

[13] William. H. Cook, *The Physiomedical Dispensatory* (Wm. H. Cook, 1869), 481. https://www.henriettes-herb.com/eclectic/cook/index.html [Ed.]

[14] As noted in footnotes above, regarding Boneset, Borage and Comfrey, please keep up to date on the research and debates around the safety of plants that contain pyrrolizidine alkaloids. [Ed.]

Culpeper's[15] indication for Comfrey, old coughs, coughs which have been around so long they've got their Zimmer frame, it's brilliant for that. The Leechbook of Bald[16] recommends Elecampane and Comfrey for a dry cough. My favourite recipe actually is Elecampane, Orange peel and Cinnamon as a decoction, it's very tasty and great for coughs. We usually like to add a syrup for coughs, you might add honey. I say to patients, "What happens is, if you add the stickiness then it goes down slowly and it sends its healing out into the lungs as it does it, so you need that going down slowly."

Elfshot

Inula helenium, Elecampane, Horseheal, Scabwort, Elf Dock. Elf Dock because it's the broad leaf plant which you use for people who are elf-shot, a well-known prescription for elfshot disease. I think of elfshot conditions as people wasting away with no obvious cause. When I first started treating chronic fatigue it struck me as that, because people look healthy, they look OK but they're wasting away. So, having read that, I started thinking that they're probably elfshot. One of the Saxon ways of diagnosing elfshot was to get the medicine man or the medicine woman, the person who knew most about these things, the Seer, to look at the person's aura, and you can see, what happens if you get elfshot is the elves shoot arrows into you and it makes invisible holes in your aura, and your energy drains out of the hole. And, apparently if you look into the hole, if you can see the hole you can see through it to the other world. I haven't managed that yet, even with a magnifying glass. It's quite easy to upset an elf, the Saxon word for good manners translates as "elf manners", elves have a way of being in the world, they have a very strict view about how you should be in the world, be with nature. And, of course, human beings do not do that, we're very slapdash and untidy and I think that's how you upset the elves.

---

[15] Culpeper, *Culpeper's Complete Herbal*, 76. [Ed.]

[16] Thomas Oswald Cockayne et al., *Leechdoms, Wortcunning, and Starcraft of Early England. Being a Collection of Documents, for the Most Part Never before Printed, Illustrating the History of Science in This Country before the Norman Conquest* (Longman, Green, Longman, Roberts, and Green, 1864), 59. https://archive.org/details/leechdomswortcun02cock/page/n7/mode/2up. [Ed.]

One of the recipes in the Leechbook[17] is for elf disease: take incense, holy salt, three heads of Garlic, well that's going to cure everybody isn't it, root of Enchanter's Nightshade and Elecampane, and then you take it into church, and you say mass over it, presumably in pre-Christian times they had Pagan rituals. But, you do a nice little ritual with it. Take these, a cup of milk with holy water dropped into it three times and drink as hot as you can bear, eating three bits of Enchanter's Nightshade at the same time. And also smoke the house with Elecampane on burning embers.

Do you know Enchanter's Nightshade? You do, jolly good. Really beautiful. It's a Fuchsia, you can see, can't you? In that family, very, very common in woodland around me, probably around you as well. It's often used for, the Saxon word for enchant, according to Cockayne, the Saxon word for Enchanter's Nightshade is "Elf Foam". So, it was much used in recipes for magical problems, what we might nowadays call psychiatric problems, along with the Elecampane. Elf, the word "elf" actually means shining one, that's what it means. And, actually, I don't know if you've ever come across this at twilight in the woods, it shines, and I think that's maybe where it got its name. I don't know.

It's quite horrible

I found that both the water soluble and the oil soluble fractions of Elecampane show immune strengthening activity, which suggests that the popular medieval recipe of Elecampane cooked in chicken stock is probably a really good way of doing it, because you're going to get the water soluble and the oil soluble constituents aren't you? I did try that, it's quite horrible.

Ephedra (*Ephedra sinica*)

Take ten students

I was taught that Ephedra tincture was very unlikely to raise blood pressure due to the balance of beta- and alpha-adrenergic alkaloids, but some doubt remains amongst students and new practitioners, so we

---

[17] Thomas Oswald Cockayne et al., *Leechdoms, Wortcunning, and Starcraft of Early England*, 347–349. [Ed.]

carried out an experiment. We took ten students, measured their BP and pulse, gave them thirty drops of Ephedra tincture—1:5 dried herb tincture in 25% alcohol—and waited ten minutes then repeated pulse and BP. One student's pulse went up a little, one student's BP went up a little and two student's BPs went down a little, and the rest were unaffected. There were no hypertensive students in the group.

Fennel (*Foeniculum vulgare*)
It tells us quite a lot

Got one of my favourite quotes here about Fennel, from Hildegard von Bingen. Hildegard von Bingen said of Fennel, "It forces the spirits back into the right balance of joyfulness."[18] I love that, don't you? That tells us something about Fennel, doesn't it? It tells us quite a lot about Hildegard actually, doesn't it.

Figwort (*Scrophularia nodosa* and *S. aquatica*)
The King's evil and a great hope for Charles

We have two common Figworts here. *Scrophularia nodosa* seems to me to be very like the Chinese species. It grows in woods and has hard, black nodules on its roots, hence the use for hard, black nodules, of most use in the upper body. Water Figwort, *S. aquatica*, also called Water Betony (after the shape of its leaves), grows in damp soil and does that thing that many marsh plants do—spreads by rhizomes, creeping along as the land dries. We use this mainly for lymphatic congestion with heavy water retention in the lower body. Both species are useful as fresh leaf dressings for skin inflammations, such as damp eczema.

---

[18] I have been unable to find a source for this exact quote, with the closest being that Fennel "brings humans a sense of joyfulness." Wighard Strehlow, *Hildegard of Bingen's Spiritual Remedies* (Rochester, Vt: Healing Arts Press, 2002), 240. Of course, Christopher may have had access to other sources/translations. I also think that Christopher's love of the quote that he found tells us something about Christopher, as much as it tells us something about Hildegard, including his embrace of the many apparent tensions in herbal medicine, to the point where they soften into something entangled rather than binary. Being forced into joyfulness sounds rather enticing. I imagine that Christopher and Hildegard would have got on very well over a cup of herbal tea and a slice of cake made with spelt, cinnamon and nutmeg, key ingredients in her pharmacopoeia. Maybe they are doing just that, right now. [Ed.]

I like to tell the students the story of scrophula (TB of the lymph nodes with persistent oozing sores) and King Edward the Confessor who liked to do the hands-on healing "in the name of Jesus" (very popular in those days), especially for nasty, weeping sores—hence the name "King's evil". The last English King to do that was Charles I. Charles II refused outright—he probably thought it would spoil his lace cuffs. Charles II was also an amateur scientist so maybe he thought the whole thing unscientific and he was famously bled to death by his doctors, in a spirit of scientific competition no doubt! We have great hopes of Charles III, if he ever gets to be so. I'm sure he will be only too happy to practice alternative healing on the oozing sores of his subjects.[19]

Fly Agaric (Amanita muscaria)

A loss of scale

Rudolph the red-nosed reindeer ate Fly Agaric. It gave him muscular strength enough to leap and fly and turned his nose red, via cholinergic actions on the neuromuscular junction and on vasodilation. Fly Agaric is not a noticeably poisonous herb. As to toxicity, reports in the literature and 1960s experience show ten fruiting bodies are safe—but a caution is needed here as the amount of active ingredients varies a great deal. Using it in drop doses is effective as only very small doses are needed. Typically, I am using less than half a fruiting body a day. The constituents do not accumulate in the body. They are water soluble and easily excreted in the urine. Looking through my sources—mostly pamphlets from the '60s—the commonest method of taking the herb seems to be to simply dry the cap, roll it up and swallow it.

A quick look through ethnobotanical sources suggests that the actions of the fungus are very consistent, namely a feeling of strength and,

---

[19] Charles III made it to the throne after Christopher's passing. So far, there are no proclamations from the Palace about any such hands-on healing being practiced by Charles III, even if he has been a long-time supporter of complementary medicine, and his mum was a patient of homeopathic physicians and reputedly carried a leather kit of remedies with her on her travels. Of course, Charles III has recently publicly announced his own cancer, with this openness potentially being a healing of sorts. I remember being told that Christopher met Prince Charles once when taking a group of students to the Duchy farm at Highgrove, telling the future monarch stories about Fly Agaric, possibly the ones that you will find below. That I would like to have seen. I really hope it's true. If not, it should be. [Ed.]

on higher doses, sleep with a series of visions as if traveling through time or space. I find it most useful at helping me maintain a state between wakefulness and sleep for long periods. In such a state, dreaming visions come with great clarity and force. There is often a loss of scale as in any dreaming practice as, of course, in Alice in Wonderland.

There is only one known case of death from Fly Agaric, but quite a few people get very sick from eating raw fungi. Hospital treatment for those who abuse the "herb" includes supportive measures, gastric lavage, activated charcoal and possibly anticholinergic drugs. The trick with any case of suspected fungi poisoning is to go to A&E fast and take some of the fungi with you. There was a recent case of a young man in Poland with a long history of mental illness. He was admitted to A&E in a coma but recovered totally in three days with conservative treatment.

Panther caps contain the same chemicals but at higher levels and should be avoided. They are possibly fatal. They are easily told by their brown caps. The common British Fly Agaric type always has red caps with a thin layer of yellow under the cap. It cannot be confused. Never eat a brown Agaric with no spots! It could be a Death Cap. A case of Death Cap poisoning has been reported as being successfully treated by chewing Milk Thistle seeds, taking the patient to hospital for follow up care.[20]

We could expect no less

Mrs Grieve[21] mentions Fireweed (Rosebay Willowherb) as being added to Fly Agaric in Siberia, which is the reason I first used that combination. She also mentions its use as an antispasmodic in lung complaints.

Biochemically speaking, Fly Agaric is cholinergic, which explains the feeling of great strength and lightness we used to find when chewing the skins on fungus forays. It is also a notable vasodilator and excellent for keeping the cold off during nights in the forest. I assume the common symptom of nausea also comes from this cholinergic activity,

---

[20] In the USA, an extract of Milk Thistle, silibinin, has become part of the Santa Cruz Protocol for Death Cap mushroom poisoning. This was pioneered by a family doctor, Dr Todd Mitchell, who learnt this from European medical practice. He describes himself as having "one foot out of the mainstream". [Ed.]

[21] Maud Grieve, *A Modern Herbal*, vol. 2 (1931; repr., Dover Publications, 1971), 848. Please also see Rosebay Willowherb, below. [Ed.]

which is possibly the main reason for adding Fireweed. It might also be to enhance the effects of the fungus.

Anyway, I have tried the Fly Agaric with and without Fireweed and have found the latter method more gentle. It is most likely that the tannins in the Rosebay delay the uptake of alkaloids. Sloe gin is also very astringent. The astringent/mucilaginous actions probably also reduce gut griping.

Christopher Hobbs has more details of chemistry, preparations, etc. in his *Medicinal Mushrooms* book[22]. The biochemistry is complex (well, it is a medicinal "herb", we could expect no less).

True of all herbs

Spiritually speaking it is a guide to the other world and hence of great use to the Shaman. It is important when using it this way to ask a clear question first, so it knows what to look out for to help you. It is also important to clearly ask its help and be respectful and listen to it. Don't take it or give it to a patient if it says no. You must approach this herb for yourself first, but that is true of all herbs.

Garlic (Allium sativum)

The simplest solution

My favourite story about that concerns the husband of a patient of mine who used to bring her up to see me. And he wouldn't come in himself of course because he's a man and men never get ill, it's a well-known fact. And one day when I was showing her out, he said to me, "I've got a problem I wouldn't mind a bit of help with," (for nothing). "I love walking, I walk all the time and just lately I've found that when I go for a walk over the Heath, I get about a quarter of the distance I used to get and I start getting pains in my calves and I can't walk any further, I have to stop." So, I said, "Do you smoke?" He said, "Oh yeah, I smoke thirty, forty cigarettes a day." So, I said, "Ah, that's intermittent claudication." That's a nice word isn't it—intermittent claudication—it makes me think of all sorts of jolly little pictures of Claude. And, I said, "Well, what you've got to do, of course, is give up smoking." He said,

---

[22] Christopher Hobbs, *Medicinal Mushrooms* (Botanica Press, 1996). Christopher Hobbs also has a newer publication that readers might be interested in: *Christopher Hobbs's Medicinal Mushrooms: The Essential Guide* (Storey Publishing, LLC, 2021). [Ed.]

"Oh no, I'm not going to give up smoking, I've only got two pleasures in life, smoking and walking long walks." Well, he wasn't going to take many herbs, so I said, "The simplest solution I can think of is just take lots of Garlic", because if we give him lots of Garlic at least it'll help him live a few years longer. "So, just take a lot of Garlic and maybe it'll help, maybe it won't help". He came back a few weeks later with his wife and he said, "That's brilliant stuff that Garlic. I walked the other day, I walked right across the heath no problem at all, as far as I ever walked and I haven't had to give up smoking."

A little pipe

I suppose the main indication for Garlic is arteriosclerosis, hardening of the arteries, blockage of the arteries. We could just give it to anybody that we suspected of circulatory problems. I usually try and assess the tone of the arteries, feeling them, do you do that test? If you occlude the artery at the wrist or any handy artery, just press it and stop the blood flowing there you shouldn't be able to feel anything on the distal side, on the furthest side away from the heart because you've stopped the blood flowing, you shouldn't be able to feel the artery at all, it should be soft and not feel it. If you can still feel the artery there like a little pipe there then there's deposits in the artery.

Garlic addresses that

The other thing I use Garlic for, it's I think the second major killer these days in modern society, it's diabetes and Garlic is very useful for diabetes, firstly because the main immediate problem from diabetes is the troubles with the circulatory system, the poor circulation, high blood pressure, tendency to the circulation blocking up, and Garlic addresses that. Also Garlic's one of the single most effective remedies for lowering blood sugar. I find it really useful with diabetics for whatever reason their blood sugar's suddenly shot up to bring it down again very quickly, just eat a lot of Garlic.

Appropriates to the human

Garlic boiled up in milk for coughs. A little bit of honey. They'd say in the old days that, two reasons for boiling the Garlic in the milk, firstly it softens the Garlic, secondly that if you're dealing with phlegmatic complaints, you put the Garlic in a phlegmatic substance like milk and what happens is the milk sidles up to the phlegm, which looks at it and thinks, "Oh there's a friendly substance" and says, "Come in!" and then the Garlic goes, "Whoosh, gotcha!" That's how you do that. Appropriates to the human, I'd say.

Ginkgo (Ginkgo biloba)

How Ginkgo leaves got their shape

Listen to the story of how the Ginkgo leaves got their shape. In the beginning, Ginkgo trees had huge leaves, hand-shaped like those on Plane trees. And like the Plane leaves, they were tough and pretty much inedible. The Ginkgo tree had grown those leaves in order to avoid being eaten by the dinosaurs that roamed the earth at that time. Those dinosaurs were big and growing bigger. Aeon by aeon they had grown longer and longer necks so they could reach the leaves on the highest edible trees. In the end their necks were so long that the blood could hardly reach their heads, their brains were deprived of oxygen and they couldn't think straight. Soon, the great Jurassic plains were covered with dozy dinosaurs, standing around waving their long, long necks and trying to remember how to move their feet—well on their way to extinction.

One day, a very small dinosaur with misshapen teeth found itself standing in the shade of a Ginkgo tree and so hungry that it was tempted to try and eat those big, tough leaves. So big and tough were those leaves that our dinosaur could only chew off the ends, leaving just the base of each leaf, and each chewed off leaf had a notch in the end where one of the dinosaur's teeth stuck out. As it chewed the leaves the dinosaur found that it could think more clearly. The blood was starting to get to its brain! It remembered how to move its feet! A great feeling of love and gratitude for the tree grew in our dinosaur's heart and it gave that tree a big, warm hug. The Ginkgo tree smiled to itself in that secret place where trees smile and its leaves turned pale yellow in joy. From that day to this, the Ginkgo tree has grown sweet, tender leaves, each baring a notch in the end in memory of its friendship with that dinosaur. It makes me wonder how the new relationship between Ginkgos and humans will change the shape of us both.

Balances the immediate effect

I was sort of thinking that the much renowned headaches come from the high flavonoid content. The immediate effect of flavonoids is vasodilation, with a sudden rush of blood to the head. Perhaps exacerbated in students? Choleric students will often go quite red in the face during Ginkgo tea tasting for example. The long-term effects are to improve circulation in general, which balances the immediate effect. Thus, headaches can often be circumvented by starting with a low dose and gradually increasing it.

Clottiness

My understanding is that the clotting process is complicated and prolonged—in biochemical terms—and that herbs, or other substances, could interact with that process at different stages and thus have different, and unsuspected, degrees of end results. It should not be a problem since patients on warfarin should be having regular blood tests anyway, even the notoriously parsimonious UK NHS can be persuaded to check INR on a regular basis.

Perhaps my all-time, for many reasons, favourite patient, is a case in point. She has a genetic blood clotting disorder and has been on warfarin for many years following a couple of pulmonary emboli. Nothing I have given her has affected her INR—including Meadowsweet, Yarrow, Garlic and essential fatty acids, all at high doses. Indeed, we tried, at her request, to reduce her dependence on warfarin by adding Ginkgo standardised extract tablets to her regime—28.8 mg Ginkgo flavonoids per tablet. The dose mentioned by Mills and Bone is up to 30 mg per day, although they mention that "recent clinical trials have used twice this dose for some applications."[23] Even three tablets a day made no difference to her INR and we gave up the attempt, for the time being. The only things that have ever affected her blood clottability were infections, stress, broccoli and brandy. I reach the

---

[23] Kerry Bone and Simon Mills, *Principles and Practice of Phytotherapy: Modern Herbal Medicine*. (Edinburgh Churchill Livingstone, Elsevier, 2000), 404. In their second edition, published in 2013, the recommended "typical" daily dose reflects this increase in dosages that have been used in some clinical trials. Kerry Bone and Simon Mills, *Principles and Practice of Phytotherapy: Modern Herbal Medicine* (Edinburgh: Churchill Livingstone, 2013), 597. [Ed.]

conclusion, validated by much research, that the most important point for people on warfarin is not to change their diet or lifestyle drastically.

On the other hand, I treated a patient taking warfarin as a preventative against stroke from cardiac arrhythmia with reasonably ordinary doses of Meadowsweet, and this did affect her INR. But then she didn't have a blood clotting disorder, simply a turbulent blood flow with a consequent increased tendency to "normal" blood clotting. I reach the conclusion, based on this and other cases, that patients on warfarin, without any demonstrated actual clotting dysfunction should be treated more cautiously than those with a pre-existing tendency to clottiness. This seems congruent with basic vitalistic principles.

I have misgivings about Ginkgo leaf as a herbal medicine, anyway. This is a remedy without significant traditional use and one which is consistently used at near pharmaceutical doses. To my mind, not a candidate for good herbal medicine. I remember herbalists being asked some time ago for prescriptions they had used with Ginkgo. All the prescriptions also contained Hawthorn. Now, using a sweet synergy in this way could well be good herbal medicine.

Goat's Rue (*Galega officinalis*)

Feeling better

I have used Galega for a long time. Some say that it probably improves pancreatic function and I believe it does so. I often use the tea as an adjunct to adaptogens. People report feeling better and having better sugar control on the tea, even people on insulin, although not such good results for autoimmune diabetes. I have used it extensively for helping people control diabetes and reactive hypoglycaemia and occasionally for helping milk production, although usually as part of a formula addressing the mother's underlying problems. One suggestion was to use the standard "keep alkaloids low technique", i.e., pick well before flowering. I almost always use it as a tea, picked from the back of a local park when it is looking really green and healthy, and well before flowering. It's a nice drinking tea.

Golden Seal (*Hydrastis canadensis*), Barberry (*Berberis vulgaris*), Mahonia (*Berberis aquifolium*)

I try my best

I was privileged to see a bed of Golden Seal in September. It spreads across the woodland floor, just under the surface and tells of its use in solidifying surfaces, which is pretty much how I use it. The BHP[24] says it stimulates smooth muscle and is therefore contraindicated in hypertension and pregnancy. All its yellow parts were hidden, which suggests that it is a herb that might have unexpected actions on a deep level. The fruit was red and unexpectedly sweet. As to cooling, I tend to think of its use for damp heat being more rooted in the drying aspect of the herb and, of course, clearing heat does not necessarily imply that the herb is cold only that it appropriates to heat. At the moment I still use a little Golden Seal for intractable cases of gastrointestinal mucus congestion and topically for infected ulcers, usually with Gotu Kola and Cedarwood oil. They heal really well, usually with very little scarring. As my partner says, "What would you expect from a herb called Seal?"

Berberis vulgaris, which is quite widely used over here, is given as contraindicated in pregnancy only. The yellowness of this plant is somewhat hidden but is implicit in its flowers. Culpeper[25] refers to Barberry as under Mars, i.e., hot and dry, and says it cleanses the body of choler by sympathy.

Berberis aquifolium is given no contraindications. The yellowness of this plant runs strongly just under the bark and bursts forth in those gloriously scented flowers. It is a straightforward plant and much easier to use. My teacher used this strong to mild grouping according to the constitution of the individual, but she would never use any of them without adding Dandelion root as well. I suppose the lesson is always to pick your herbs by the constitution of the patient. I try my best. Do you know the *B. aquifolium* stamen jumping trick, as taught to me by a beekeeper? Touch the stigma of an unfertilized flower with the point of a thorn and the stamens jump at you—no doubt mistaking you for a very large bee. Keeps the students, and passing tourists, amused for hours.

---

[24] British Herbal Medicine Association. Scientific Committee, *British Herbal Pharmacopoeia, 1983* (London: British Herbal Medicine Association, 1983), 114. [Ed.]

[25] Culpeper, *Culpeper's Complete Herbal*, 22. [Ed.]

Greater Celandine (Chelidonium majus)
If you give enough of it

I suppose Celandine must be poisonous if you give enough of it. Mrs Grieve[26], who is the best source of information on practical poisoning, doesn't cite any episodes, but then I suppose it isn't a very appetising herb, unlike Water Hemlock, for example. The juice is certainly acrid and burns somewhat, but I have used glycerine extracts of the fresh plant for cataracts many times without problems (diluted 1:3 or 1:4 with water). It is also excellent for corns and bunions. A little care must be applied when using it for warts on soft skin, but I have never had trouble on hard skin. I have tried it a few times on carcinoma, but patients usually give up early and go for the operation. It shares many alkaloids with Bloodroot (*Sanguinaria canadensis*).

The British Herbal Pharmacopeia[27] dose is up to 6 ml daily for an FE (1:1). I use a 1:5 fresh plant tincture, which would be equivalent to a 1:30 dried plant tincture, if it is possible to make an equivalence here. I have used this at 10 to 20 ml daily for liver cancer, sometimes with success. King's American Dispensatory[28] gives a tincture (three ounces to one pint) dose of one to fifteen drops for the "specific purposes for which it is now employed" of "full, pale, sallow tongue and mucous membranes; skin pale and sallow, sometimes greenish." They also give Scudder as using even smaller doses (ten drops in a cup of water, use 15 ml every three or four hours). What I glean from all this is that the herb works best when used in small doses.

Hawthorn (*Crataegus* spp.)
Takes longer, of course

As I see it, Hawthorn is basically a blood vessel trophorestorative, and especially an arterial/arteriole trophorestorative, relaxing and improving tissue strength and improving blood flow—being applicable to the heart only in so far as that organ may be considered to be an

---

[26] Grieve, *A Modern Herbal*. [Ed.]

[27] British Herbal Medicine Association, *British Herbal Pharmacopoeia*, 62. [Ed.]

[28] Harvey Wickes Felter and John Uri Lloyd, *King's American Dispensatory* (Cincinnati: Ohio Valley Co., 1898), https://www.henriettes-herb.com/eclectic/kings/intro.html. [Ed.]

enlarged artery. Priest and Priest[29] give, "increases and sustains action of heart and arterioles, with principal influence on the myocardium. Improves coronary circulation, restores myocardial reserve and regulates disturbances of rhythm ... Individual Indications: myocardial degeneration and/or coronary sclerosis in elderly—with sufficient Cactus/Capsicum to sustain function."

Priest and Priest were in the straight line of the British Physiomedical tradition and give the best explanation of the philosophy and practical therapeutics of that tradition. The elder Priest ran the school for the National Institute of Medical Herbalists for many years. He stopped taking an active part in Institute affairs when the pseudoscientific constituent chemistry approach started to take hold. I believe that Physiomedicalism is the best route to a modern approach to herbal medicine—uniting traditional and current orthodox approaches to medicine.

Trophorestoring is a nourishing, i.e., long-term, action. As has been pointed out, restorative herbs may be more active than restoring in the short term. I have noted that with Hawthorn, and with other high flavonoid herbs, the vasodilator action kicks in quickly leading to a quick drop in BP in susceptible (usually asthenic)[30] individuals or headaches in susceptible (usually sthenic)[31] individuals. The restorative effect takes longer, of course. If I had a bad reaction to Hawthorn from a patient then I would be tempted to drop the dose right down and continue—of course, I may simply decide that there are more suitable herbs. My teacher, who had been taught by Priest, said that, "If you are sure that a herb is the right one for your patient and you get an untoward reaction, then half the dose and continue."

Addressing fear

I don't think of Hawthorn as a nervine but I do agree that it lends strength to a nervine mixture—as I see it, by addressing fear. The arteries are the conduit of the Vital Spirit. Arterial restoratives ease the flow

---

[29] A.W. Priest and L.R. Priest, *Herbal Medication: A Clinical and Dispensary Handbook*, 90–91, (The C.W. Daniel Company Ltd, 2000). [Ed.]

[30] In Physiomedical thinking, asthenic individuals have over-relaxed tissues, often presenting with poor circulation, coldness, a build-up of metabolic waste and tissue atrophy. [Ed.]

[31] On the other hand, sthenic individuals demonstrate an over-reactive state, often presenting with tension and tight muscles, as well as inflammation and pain. [Ed.]

Start low

My general inclination with Hawthorn and severe heart problems is to start low, say 15 gtt t.d.s.[32] and work up. Dr Jennings[33] recommended 4 to 8 gtt q.d.s.[34] This level of dose was common amongst British Physiomedicalists of my teacher's generation. I haven't had any specific problems with Hawthorn. The whole area of orthodox treatment and diagnosis seems very tricky to me. Very often patients have the full range of tests and no clear results that make sense to me anyway. I wonder, for example, about their use of cardiac glycosides when Lily of the Valley can often be seen to work better, at much lower doses. Of course, I usually use this herb with Hawthorn and then we have synergy, although I have used it as a simple at 5 gtt as needed for occasional tachycardia.

Agree in no time at all

A student was wanting to do a dissertation on Hawthorn, and you probably know in Chinese herbal medicine, Hawthorn berries are used for food stagnation, for not digesting your food properly, for food getting stuck, and in English Medicine, European Medicine, it is mostly used for the heart. And how come? Well, of course, they're different species, so that's a start. That's maybe a clue and I tasted some, I hadn't done this before. They had some Chinese Hawthorn berries there and they're big. They're like little apples, like crab apples and they taste like crab apples, they're sour. I use crab apple leather for clearing food stagnation, do you? Wonderful, really good. So, if people tend to get their food stuck there, you just give them bits of crab apple leather to chew and that nice sour taste clears the stagnation from there and moves it on. The reason being of course is they're quite big and so they're

---

[32] The Latin abbreviation "gtt" translates as drops, and "t.d.s" as three times daily. [Ed.]

[33] Finley Ellingwood, *American Materia Medica, Therapeutics and Pharmacognosy* (Ellingwood's Therapeutist, 1919), 218. https://wellcomecollection.org/works/jt4unq8f/items. Also available at the Henriette Kress's website: https://www.henriettes-herb.com/eclectic/ellingwood/index.html [Ed.]

[34] The Latin abbreviation "q.d.s." translates as four times daily.

more fleshy, so they've got more of the fruit acids in. It's chemistry this. Whereas our Hawthorn berries are quite small, so they're mainly skin, so they've got more of the tannins, the anthocyanins, so they're much more for the circulation. So, there's a crossover thing. But just, just to resolve that issue, it was nice, just to do a little tasting. Tasting resolved that issue very quickly and clearly and easily. If ever you find yourself arguing with a herbalist, just sit down and taste the herb and you'll agree in no time at all.

The issue is redness

It seems to me that the difference between large and small Hawthorn berries is the same as the difference between Blueberries and Bilberries. In these two the ratio of blueness to flesh is higher in the smaller berries, making them more useful as medicines—and the larger more useful as food. With Crataegus species, of course, the issue is redness.

Clearing remedy

OK Hawthorn. Hawthorn, the heart remedy, yes? As you're probably aware, of course, it was totally made up by the Eclectics, wasn't it? Didn't exist before then, they invented it. In the old medical texts Hawthorn is just a minor herb used for kidney stones and maybe abdominal spasm and all of a sudden it's the major heart remedy in the universe. How did that happen? I think the Hawthorn fairy thought to itself, "I deserve more than this."

I actually think Rudolph Weiss, the German herbalist, put his finger on it really well when he said, "The main indications for Crataegus are undoubtedly degenerative conditions of the type seen commonly today."[35] The problem, of course, is what happened is that in the old days people exercised a lot, their heart diseases were different from the heart diseases we get these days and Hawthorn is more applicable to the heart disease that we get these days which is to do with congestion, especially congestion of the arteries. Hawthorn is a clearing remedy, that's the bottom line, it's got those little spines that go, "Clear! Clear! Clear!" In the old days they'd use it for clearing the digestion or clearing the kidneys, these days we use it for clearing the heart and the

---

[35] Weiss, *Herbal Medicine*, 165. [Ed.]

congestion there. That's my take on that. Hawthorn is in many ways more of an arterial remedy, it's really for the arteries. It clears and strengthens the arteries, it clears cholesterol, it strengthens arterial tone, but by doing that of course it improves the heart, because the heart has got arteries as well. Even arteries have arteries, don't they? The big ones do.

Like a good bouncer

Hawthorn is a really good example of a tonic, a restorative herb, a herb which is gentle but not weak. That's another nice thing that Rudolph Weiss says, "Don't mistake gentleness for weakness."[36] I sometimes think that herbs are like really good bouncers in a nightclub. A really good bouncer is gentle, they talk you out the door, a good bouncer doesn't go in there and start hitting people. I think a good herb is like a good bouncer, he goes into the nightclub, which is your body, and it identifies the disease, which is the person playing up and causing trouble and getting too drunk, and it just edges it out, a little bit of a nudge. That's a good herb. So, it's a restorative. I suppose the basic rule nowadays if there's anything wrong with the heart or the arteries you just chuck Hawthorn in and people will get better.

That pleased me

In many ways, it's probably the most useful herb in all sorts of ways. I remember seeing someone, it wasn't my patient, it was somebody else's patient who was dying of cancer, hadn't got long to live, he was still walking around, liver cancer and he'd just been, he'd come down to London to go to the hospital for tests and his son said, maybe he should come and see me and there wasn't anything I could really do. All I did was I gave him a bottle of Hawthorn tincture because he was complaining about his heart, in an emotional way, not in a physical way, with a few drops of Rescue Remedy in and it lifted him up, he said he hadn't felt so good for ages and ages. Hawthorn berry tincture actually. It's a great lift-up for any circumstances.

I treated somebody last year for depression, for severe depression. When I heard her family history, I wasn't surprised at all, I was actually surprised that she was still there never mind depressed. And she said, one of the symptoms she described was a feeling of emptiness, heaviness,

---

[36] Weiss, *Herbal Medicine*, 1. [Ed.]

coldness in the heart area, in the heart chakra area really and I gave her, because she was of a phlegmatic constitution, I gave her Hawthorn with a bit of Ginger in for the warming and she came back two weeks later, her depression hadn't gone, there's lots of work to do and lots of therapy to go through, but she said, "That's the first time in my entire life that I've felt normal in that area." Isn't that nice? "I really felt that there was some solidity and warmth in that area." That pleased me.

Herb Bennet, Wood Avens (Geum urbanum)

Rampant in my garden

I gather Herb Bennet each year in the early part of the season when it is in lush growth. I use it in teas and tinctures, especially as a gentle astringent for children's diarrhoea. I use the whole plant including the roots as a short decoction for diarrhoea or as a gastrointestinal astringent in general. The roots add a warming element, which the intestinal tract finds very comforting. They are also antiseptic. It is also a herb of protection, to be hung over your door or grown close to your door. It is rampant in my garden, which has damp, clay soil. Because it is so abundant, I wondered whether it was a herb that I could use. When I looked it up, I found that it was used for gut inflammation so I thought it would be particularly useful given the number of patients I see with this as a problem. I don't know much about this herb but was intrigued to learn that the roots had a Clove-like smell when dug up and that seemed to fit with the gut healing properties. It contains ellagitannins, which are soluble in both alcohol and water. Ellagitannins are being investigated for possible therapeutic benefits in the treatment of irritable bowel syndrome and ulcerative colitis. It seems to be specific for ulcerative colitis. Taken as a decoction in the spring, Herb Bennet acts as a purifier and removes obstructions of the liver.

Slightly different direction

Herb Bennet is a gut astringent similar to *Agrimonia eupatoria* and *Geranium maculatum*. What might be the differences between these three? Herb Bennet, used with the root, is the most warming and best for cold conditions or empty heat conditions such as colitis and after a bout of food poisoning. *Agrimonia eupatoria*, on the other hand, has a slight bitter edge and is useful for the liver, so I use it a great deal for food sensitivities and leaky gut. It is also brilliant for people who feel zonked out after eating. And *Geranium maculatum* is the best of the three for toning the bladder, so its appropriation would be lower down. Julian Barker[37] makes the point that, even though astringents all have the same actions they each come from a slightly different direction. So, he suggests always using a combination. Gastrointestinal astringents work best as teas.

Hops (*Humulus lupulus*)

Hop babies

The situation is complex due to the different activity of oestrogen receptors. I did have one female patient who had stopped taking Hops as a sedative because they made her breasts grow. She challenged this twice and was convinced. I use Hops often as a sedative and I haven't noticed this in other patients—but then I am using quite small amounts. It is possible that the "anti-testosterone" activity in men is due, at least partly, to pelvic nerve sedation. Melancholic men find that Hops, including beer, induces depression and thus lowers sexual interest. I have seen this effect a few times at close hand. I come from a Hop picking area and used to work in the fields. In my day, most picking was done from trailers simply by pulling the vines down and stripped by machine, but there was still a small amount picked by hand, by women for the best quality beers. In older times, most of the picking was done by hand by women who came down from London for a "Hop holiday". Husbands were often left at home but the male farm labourers were around. This often led to "Hop babies" which may be the original source of the idea of Hops promoting sexuality in women.

Horsetail (*Equisetum arvense*)

The minerals contribute

If we consider the pharmacology, Horsetail contains a saponin, flavonoids, alkaloids including nicotine, sterols, and a wide range of minerals including silica and zinc. The minerals contribute. They are not the whole of the herb, but they point to a building and strengthening action as well as the generally understood cleansing activity. It seems to improve mineral metabolism in general. I don't think it reasonable to categorise it

---

[37] Barker, *The Medicinal Flora of Britain & Northwest Europe*. [Ed.]

as a tonic. Rebalancing might be a better category—the building action being rooted in the rebalancing of underlying metabolism.

I don't see how Horsetail can be classified as an anti-inflammatory except in local use where the anti-inflammatory action is part of its overall wound healing action. I have used it to strengthen hair, to improve lung efficiency in emphysema and to repair damage to the urinary tract. It is also used to strengthen bones and as a strengthening nail polish. It is a good antifungal and may be included in topical treatments for fungal infections of the nail bed. The tincture seems to work well enough in all the above conditions. I have not used it as a powder. Since it is often used to scour pans, this method of administration doesn't seem suitable.

Russian traditional use is to strengthen the hair. There is a Russian folk tale concerning an old woman whose land was so poor it grew nothing but Horsetail. In desperation, she appealed to the grandmother Horsetail plant for help. It turned into a beautiful princess with long flowing hair and everywhere she walked ermine sprung from her footsteps. I am not quite sure how the ermine got there but they solved the old woman's financial problems.

I am happy with the tincture

The Galenic classification is cold and dry in the second degree. This does not necessarily imply an overall cooling action, but rather an appropriation to cold, dry tissues such as hair, skin and bones. The dominant virtue of the herb is its dryness. It is not generally used on its own except when only that dryness is needed. It would seem that the silica is not particularly well extracted in the tincture and some people here recommend a four-hour decoction with the addition of a little sugar in order to maximise silica extraction, or the use of a juice—yes, you can get juice from Horsetail, especially the sterile fronds and young plants. I used to do this and I might again but for the time being I am happy with the tincture.

Juniper (*Juniperus communis*)

Black furry shapes

A few years ago, I treated a young couple, very much in love. They got married, moved into a new flat and after a while started arguing with each other and shouting at each other all the time. And after some time, the lady next door said to them, "I hope you don't mind me saying this but the previous couple that came here were shouting at each other all the time." Patients tell you anything don't they, that's what's so nice about herbal medicine, patients say all sorts of things, and then they say, like this couple did, "Why am I telling you that?" And I said, "Well, obviously the thing to do, there's bad vibes in that house, as we say. We need to smudge it and you'll smudge it with Juniper, Juniper berries or Juniper oil on a piece of charcoal, and you open the front door and you stand by the front door and see what happens." And she did, and she said, "You know what happened? All these little black furry shapes came rushing out of the front door."[38]

Kelp (including *Fucus vesiculosus*)

Tip people over

I was taught that Kelp has an alterative action specific to resolving swellings. Priest[39], for example, taught its use in hydrocele of the scrotum. My teacher made up a Kelp cream for swollen joints. Goitres respond to Kelp but be careful using it in non-goitre underactive thyroid. I have found, in many such cases, that small amounts have a dramatic effect, sometimes any more than 10 ml a week will tip people over into hyperactivity, presumably there is a sensitivity involved. Following a tip in Peter Holmes[40], I have used Damiana for underactive thyroid people of all kinds and found it very helpful.

Lady's Mantle (*Alchemilla vulgaris, A. mollis*)

The lady in the sweet shop

Let's talk about Lady's Mantle. Here's a Lady's Mantle leaf I picked from my garden. It's even got, courtesy of the weather, raindrops on it, not dew, but raindrops. And, of course, not that magical water

---

[38] If you have watched the film "My Neighbour Totoro", you may have seen these shapes too, as Soot Sprites. If you haven't watched it, there's a treat in store for you. [Ed.]

[39] Given that Christopher says that Priest "taught" this application, he may have come across this in his studies at the School of Herbal Medicine, where A.W. Priest taught before Christopher was a student. I have been unable to find any mention of this is Priest and Priest, *Herbal Medication*, or in papers published by A.W. Priest—see footnote to Seeds, "Tradition and direct knowing". [Ed.]

[40] Peter Holmes, *The Energetics of Western Herbs: A Materia Medica Integrating Western and Chinese Herbal Therapeutics*, vol. 1 (Boulder, Colo.: Snow Lotus Press, 2007), 340. This two-volume set has now been republished by Aeon Books as a single volume. [Ed.]

that Lady's Mantle secretes all by itself even on a hot dry day. This is *mollis, Alchemilla mollis,* which is the commonest Lady's Mantle in people's gardens here. Widely grown as undercover in parks and gardens. It's a Turkish species. Doesn't make any difference, any species can be used. Well, this is just a little bit softer and furrier, that's all, but the properties are the same. I love the way, let's have a look, closer look, I love the way the edge is cut, crimped very, very, very carefully, and then the delicate silver line right round. And of course, the whole thing is pleated. I do think the Lady's Mantle fairies must be a bit obsessive to go to all that bother. The flowers are very simple, but then if you're obsessive I think simple is better, you can make it tidier and neater.

Right, Lady's Mantle stories. My favourite Lady's Mantle story. Some years ago, when I was just starting out as a herbalist, an Indian lady in the sweet shop, not that I ever go into the sweet shop, of course, called me over and said, "I hear you're a herbalist, do you have anything for heavy periods?" I thought to myself, well, it's a good way to get the punters in, give them some herbal tea, tell them if it doesn't work as well as it should do, then you've got to come and make an appointment to see me. Gave her a big bag of Lady's Mantle and waited. A couple of months later she called me round from behind a lamp post in the street, she was a bit shy, and said, "Could that herb have stopped my periods completely?" and being a new herbalist, I had a panic, I thought, "What have I done? What have I done?" and I asked a question you should always ask in those situations, "Could you be pregnant?" And she said, "I couldn't possibly be pregnant, my husband and I have been trying for eight years." But, she was. Unfortunately, the reason for the heavy bleeding was a fibroid, and the baby sat on the fibroid during the whole pregnancy, and the fibroid sat on a nerve, so she was in considerable pain. But then, she had the baby and forgot all about that. And I got invited to the christening. That was nice.

I use that term with affection and respect

I've use Lady's Mantle a lot for women who can't get pregnant when there's no particular reason, no obvious reason. I've used it a lot for women who wanted to have their babies close together, so you give them the Lady's Mantle straight after the other one. And that's worked. I even used it once for a young athlete who didn't want to have her period on the day of a big meet and her period was due then. I said,

"Take the Lady's Mantle now", it was about a month before, "and you won't have a period", and she didn't. I suppose that's psychosomatic, that's not the right word, is it? Placebo effect, that's a good word. Everyone that takes Lady's Mantle remarks on how kind and gentle it is, how happy it makes them feel. Even my more mad patients, I use that term with affection and respect, I was treating a slightly mad patient recently, trying to get her periods synchronised with the moon, she's into astrology and all that sort of thing, and the Mugwort hadn't worked, which was my basic strategy, so I thought we'll try the Lady's Mantle. Didn't work at all, I said "It hasn't worked, try some of this", and she said, "No, I'd like to keep on with the Lady's Mantle because it makes me feel really, really good."

Mainstay

Lady's Mantle is my mainstay for fibroids and endometriosis and pelvic congestion, combined with Yarrow, that combination, I must have used tons of that tea, Lady's Mantle and Yarrow. For inflammatory conditions like endometriosis, then we use Marigold as well. And don't forget if you're treating endometriosis and inflammation of the pelvis, don't forget the Castor oil packs, it's a lot of bother, but it's definitely worth it. The Marigold of course is for tidying, clearing the lymph, calming down the inflammation. Lady's Mantle is also invaluable for erratic bleeding, menopause, you know when women will have no periods for a while and then it will flood, that will deal with that situation quite easily. The French say that Lady's Mantle is progesteronic. And you can, in some cases, use it instead of Vitex for premenstrual tension. But mostly it's used for toning the womb, and I think any hormone effect must be secondary to the effect on the womb. It affects the tissue, it's a tissue herb, and if you affect the tissues, then you affect the feedback to the endocrine system, I think that's what happens.

It worked really well

What else about Lady's Mantle? Oh yes, I had a patient a few years ago, the lady worked in the City, a banker. She was suffering from stress, which is sort of obvious, and irritable bowel, and we got those better, but she still wanted to come and see me, and she kept making up little reasons to come and see me, and in the end, I just kept making up little things for her to do. And one of the things I got for her to do, because she was a little bit spotty, was to take the dew from the Lady's Mantle, so you've got to get up at dawn, and she said, "Well, there's a park across from me and there's Lady's Mantle growing there, I'll gather the dew at dawn from there" and I said, "Wash your face in it every day for the month of May", and she did it, and it worked really well.

Not actually dew

Toning the skin, toning the spots, toning the breasts after having babies to get the breasts back into tone, a little spray, just tea in the spray, that works well. Just a magic herb really. My general theory about why it didn't work for the alchemists is because they sent their apprentices out to gather the drops that the Lady's Mantle secretes, it's not actually dew, so that they could use water in their distillation process which hadn't come from the earth or the air, and the apprentices got a bit lazy and took a bit of dew and a bit of rain water, and so that's why alchemists never ever managed to change lead into gold. Although, I suppose if they had done, they wouldn't be telling us about it, would they? OK, thank you, have fun.

Lily of the Valley (Convallaria majalis)
Disturbance of the Shen too

We are taught, over here, to use Convallaria for heart failure, specific indication tachycardia +/− arrhythmia and this is what I do and it is very good, along with Hawthorn, of course. Heart failure will always follow valve disease. Culpeper[41] used it for what Chinese medicine people will recognise as disturbance of the Shen, that is disturbance of the vital spirit (which, of course, resides in the heart) and I have used it for that too and, with Rescue Remedy, for intermittent tachycardia in patients with a history of endocarditis.

---

[41] In Chinese medicine, Shen is one of the vital substances of the body and has many translations, including "spirit", "vitality", and "mind". An anxious heart can lead to disturbed Shen, manifesting as insomnia, dream disturbed sleep, anxiety, palpitations, depression, difficulty concentrating, amongst other things. Culpeper refers to Lily of the Valley as a herb that "comforts the heart and vital spirits". See: Culpeper, *Culpeper's Complete Herbal*, 149. [Ed.]

There are no contraindications for Lily of the Valley—except for concurrent administration of Foxglove glycosides (including digitoxin), which would be silly anyway. I have, in one case, weaned a patient off digitoxin and onto Lily of the Valley, which she much preferred. I tend to use 15 ml a week and you will need that for established heart failure—or at least I do—but I was taught that you could use a lot less if you used it with Hawthorn, which is just common sense really. There is an emotional effect from even quite low doses, especially if you pick the herb in flower, *and* there is always a huge emotional component of heart problems. If I am feeling good and have good emotional nourishing then I can walk up the hill with no problem—if not, then not and so on.

Subtle aspects of bitterness

Lily of the Valley contains cardiac glycosides, so it's not a gentle restorative tonic herb, it's a herb for irregular heartbeat and palpitations, for tachycardia, for fast heartbeat. I brought some in with me, have you ever, anybody not used it? I brought a bottle, so you can have a taste. It's one of my all-time favourite remedies. You've seen it growing? It's even a nice colour isn't it look, there we are, have a go. It has that nice quality of bitterness. One of the things about being a herbalist isn't it, is appreciating all the different subtle aspects of bitterness isn't it, that your patients don't really appreciate, they just say, "Oh that's nasty!" It's a particular type of bitterness, a sort of certain solid bitterness which appropriates in Chinese medicine to the heart, it plays to the heart.

It doesn't hold like Hawthorn does

So, Lily of the Valley is our, in Europe anyway, is our preferred source of cardiac glycosides. It's really good, just a few drops like that will slow your heart down straight away. Maybe if anybody would like to get extremely worried for us? It's always handy when sick people turn up to talks, isn't it? They can get better in front of everybody's eyes. The main indication for this is heart failure, of course. So, this goes into my remedies for heart failure along with the Hawthorn. It's a quicker acting remedy than the Hawthorn, but it doesn't hold like the Hawthorn does, you have to keep doing it and keep doing it and keep doing it.

Just a little tool

I have a patient who's a great unsolved mystery to the entire universe, I think. And she has heart troubles, no doubt about it she has heart troubles, has all sorts of problems with the heart, heart failure symptoms mostly. She's been to test after test after test after test and no one's ever found anything actually wrong with her, but everybody admits there's actual physical things going on right now. One thing that happens to her is from time to time she'll get all-of-a-sudden episodes of her heart racing, tachycardia, very, very fast, gets her really worried, a few drops of Lily of the Valley with a bit of Rescue Remedy in and she just takes three or four drops and the heart's calmed down straight away. So, just a little tool. It's nice to give people these little tools isn't it, which they can take at home. It's helpful anyway because they can treat themselves when you're not there and it's also enabling for them and the bottom line is enablement, isn't it?

Keep the heart ticking over

You've got to stay within the dosage, the maximum dose is twenty drops three times a day. That's actually a legal limit in the UK. Well, no I think the legal limit is twenty-four.[42] A one-in-five tincture, of the leaves and flowers, I like to use the flowers as well, because then they address the emotional aspect of the whole thing. Twenty drops, three times a day is the maximum I use, often less. My friend Stephen who works in the old folk's home, he always puts in just a little bit of Lily of the Valley in almost everybody's medicine. Just, general grounds, when you're getting a bit older, then it's quite a good idea just to keep the heart ticking over and just a little tiny bit, just as a reminder as it were. Irregular heartbeats, the prime indication's heart failure. Either side, or both sides at once if you like.

---

[42] The schedule 20 maximum daily dose for Lily of the Valley is 450 mg, with a maximum single dose of 150 mg. The maximum daily dose of a 1:8 tincture would therefore be 3.6 ml. As there are about 20 drops to a ml (depending on the viscosity of the tincture, size of the bore hole and even height above sea level) 60 drops would be more or less 3 ml, getting close to the maximum, and 24 drops would be 3.6 ml, hitting the nail right on the head. You can tell that Christopher had a good head for numbers, and a good head all round. [Ed.]

Lime Flowers (Tilia spp.)

Four limes

High summer and the Linden flowers are opening. First the large leafed, then the intermediate, then the small leafed, which is much planted in parks and generally easier to reach, and finally the silver Lime, which has the best and strongest scent. A bowl of silver Lime flowers in the living room will keep their scent for weeks. Only the small-leafed lime is native, so I feel blessed to live in the city where I can find all four and so never miss the season no matter how tardy.

Plenty of Linden trees around the London streets, of course, but not enough to keep the people calm. London councils have taken to planting Ginkgo trees which are very pretty but tend to be on the speedy side to be around. Still, we can tell the story of how the Ginkgo leaves got their shape.[43]

Mayweed (Anthemis cotula)

A lovely piece of disused railway line

There used to be a lovely piece of disused railway line by us, they've built a supermarket on it now. And I used to go there and pick Red Clover and Sneezewort, one of the very few places in London where Sneezewort would grow, because it was well drained with the gravel underneath the railway line. And one year, I picked Red Clover for a patient whose periods had stopped, and the Red Clover told me to pick the Mayweed that was growing next to it. So, I picked the two together, I didn't know anything about Mayweed at the time. Mayweed is an old herb for energising the womb, and that really worked, that combination. So, to nourish with the Red Clover and to energise with the Mayweed is a good herbal strategy, isn't it? They were holding hands, they were growing together, and they held my hands when they taught me. We learn from the plants.

---

[43] See, Ginkgo, *How Ginkgo leaves got their shape*, in Seeds, this volume. [Ed.]

Milk Thistle (Silybum marianum syn. Carduus marianus)

Operation put off

I am treating a schoolgirl, aged thirteen, for *petit mal*, diagnosed one year ago. She has mainly absence fits, sometimes several a day. The hospital tried a few antiepileptic drugs without much success. They are considering an operation but aren't too positive about the prospects of success. She wouldn't take my medicines, neither teas nor tinctures. Her mother noted that she was tired all the time, sleeping up to eleven hours with a tendency to run hot. She has been off school for three months. She seems a personable girl, not depressed although somewhat fed up. Her mother asked me for something for her low energy. Thinking this might well be due to the heavy load on her liver from the drugs, I gave her Milk Thistle tablets, which she took. There was some improvement in her energy so I continued with the Milk Thistle. After two months, just on Milk Thistle, her energy is improving and her fits are markedly less frequent—so much so that she has put off the operation. I am wondering if the Milk Thistle has central nervous system benefits, in addition to its other virtues. I came across a piece of research[44] comparing the herb favourably to an SSRI in treating obsessive compulsive disorders, mentioning Milk Thistle being used in Iran—presumably for psychiatric disorders.

Runs under me when I sit down

The only time I treated a racehorse was, according to its stable boy, for liver damage from a parasite. I consulted with a friend who has treated horses a few times and came up with ground Milk Thistle seed with a little Ginger given one ounce daily made up into balls with molasses. The horse then started to win races and we won a little money—not a lot since that didn't seem right but enough to give moral support as it were.

I can't resist adding Culpeper's[45] comments on Melancholy Thistle (*Cirsium heterophyllum*): "The decoction of the thistle in wine being drunk, expels superfluous melancholy out of the body, and makes a

---

[44] Mehdi Sayyah et al., "Comparison of Silybum Marianum (L.) Gaertn. with Fluoxetine in the Treatment of Obsessive–Compulsive Disorder," *Progress in Neuro-Psychopharmacology and Biological Psychiatry* 34, no. 2 (March 17, 2010): 362–65, https://doi.org/10.1016/j.pnpbp.2009.12.016. [Ed.]

[45] Culpeper, *Culpeper's Complete Herbal*, 254. [Ed.]

man as merry as a cricket; superfluous melancholy causes care, fear, sadness, despair, envy and many evils more beside; but religion teaches to wait upon God's providence, and cast our cares upon him who cares for us. What a fine thing were it if men and women could live so!"

Sow Thistle is a corruption of "soft thistle" which might give us a clue to its non-thistly nature. *Sonchus* species are also used in Tibetan medicine for their gentle liver action. They also make decent vegetables. Eaten the same way as Chicory. They are generally cooler than the prickly thistles.

Dwarf thistle is *Cirsium acaule*. It grows on our chalk downland. It has no stem and is easily missed when not in flower, especially when you are sitting down to have a well-earned rest after just walking up the downland. I strongly suspect that it lurks and waits to run under me when I sit down.

All thistle flowers make good vegetables eaten like Artichokes—i.e., the base (or unripe seeds) nibbled. They taste just like Artichokes as well. On which basis I teach that all Thistles are good for the liver. I feel backed up in this assertion by Eeyore who, like all melancholics, was in constant need of gentle liver cleansing.

Motherwort (*Leonurus cardiaca*)

Within about ten seconds

OK, Motherwort. The saying about Motherwort is, "Drink Motherwort and live to be a source of continuing astonishment and grief to waiting heirs."[46] But it's another herb if taken on a regular basis, you get a good relationship with it. Motherwort is a particularly good herb for women. Maybe this is why women live much longer, because there's all these nice herbs for helping women live longer. Not fair really, is it? Well, it probably is in the end.

We use Motherwort for protecting the heart. Motherwort lowers overactive thyroid function so it calms and protects the heart. As a simple it's a brilliant herb for irregular heartbeat. It's a good herb for high blood pressure. It relaxes the womb, it's used at birth. It's used for period pains. It's used in menopause. I gave a talk once to some herbal midwives and they said they liked to use Motherwort for helping women at any time of change. And they looked at the leaf and they

---

[46] Gabrielle Hatfield, *Memory, Wisdom, and Healing: The History of Domestic Plant Medicine* (Alan Sutton Publishing, 1999), 55. [Ed.]

showed me the leaf and said it's like a hand, a soft, furry hand. There's a nice soft, supportive hand which holds you and protects you through any time of change in your life. From when your periods start, when your periods finish, when you're dying, when you're having babies, when you change jobs, when you change relationships. It's a nice one because it supports both the womb and the heart. *Leonurus cardiaca*, supports the heart.

The first time I ever grew Motherwort I grew it in the garden and I spent the whole summer stroking it because it's really nice, soft. Not too soft, nice soft touch. And I was really looking forward to cutting it, and it flowered, I let it flower a little bit like that, so there's some seeds coming in. I cut it down, took into the kitchen, got out the moon knife and within about ten seconds my hand was reduced to a bleeding mess. And I thought, what's going on here? And I realised there's all these spiny seed capsules sticking in and I thought, that's why it's called Motherwort! Because it's a nice soft, gentle herb, but don't mess with it. l think that's logical, don't you?

Mugwort (*Artemisia vulgaris*)

Save on the cinema sort of dreaming

I think what Mugwort does for women is energise the womb, so it's particularly good when there's no energy in the womb. That's just the way I view it, obviously. I view it as energising the womb, clearing blockages and it's used for painful periods with light flow. So, it relaxes and clears and gives strength to the womb so the periods are increased. If you put Mugwort in a medicine, I think it will take the medicine to the womb.

Appropriations are the part of the body to which the herb takes most of its energy really, but the other appropriation of Mugwort is to the central nervous system. So, sometimes when you give out Mugwort to put under the pillow, people will come back to me, lots of people come back with stories about lucid dreaming and whatever, or just full colour technicolour 3D, save on the cinema sort of dreaming. Or sometimes, they just say that it kept me awake all night. And sometimes people come back and say that it wasn't good. One person, the first time this happened to me, somebody came back and said, "I dreamt of a mouse all night, it was running up and down a stalk inside my head." He looked up mouse in his dream book and it said anxiety. Now the interesting thing about this is it only ever happens to men, I've never, ever known it happen to women. And I think the reason is obvious, it's the energy, if you've got a womb then the energy is split between the womb and the central nervous system. If you haven't got a womb then the energy will go straight up into your head and if you tend, this guy was a little bit bipolar, just a little bit, if you tend to that manic persuasion, then it'll just push you along. So, it's a good strategy, take the Mugwort for a few days, just to get the feeling of the Mugwort and then, before bed, add in the herb, whichever herb you want to study and the Mugwort will guide you to the spirit of the herb in your dreams and you'll come up with all sorts of things. And you can write a book about it and make lots of money.

That's what Mugwort does

It is a herb for setting you off, setting you on the path and so if people are completely anxious, especially if people are anxious because they don't know what to do, or where to go or maybe they don't really enjoy their work but they don't know what to do about it. Then you give them Mugwort and say, "It'll set you on your path," and it will. There's quite an amazing number of herbalists that happened that way. That's a good path, isn't it? I think everyone should be a herbalist myself. It's a good path.

I never pick anything until I come across Mugwort and I carry the piece of Mugwort with me and ask it to guide me to what needs to be picked that day. So, you're thinking, "Oh I must pick Clover! I must pick Clover! I must pick Clover!" Just let it go and see what happens. And then you'll turn around and there'll be a wonderful Cramp bark or something right behind you and that's what you're picking that day. So, I'll put a piece of Mugwort next to my heart, and the Mugwort will guide me, because that's what Mugwort does.

My advertising sign

And I'll often give Mugwort to people to hang over their doorways. To protect them from evil things like, I don't know, politicians and taxmen and things of that kind. It's quite a good idea I think if you're in the healing business to have some sort of protection and hang a protection over the doorway is the first point, so people don't bring bad stuff in with them, which they do tend to do, then they don't do that. "Oh look, mummy!" a little child said last week, "Oh look mummy, there's a plant over the door." I said, "Oh yes, that's my advertising sign."

I quite often use it for psychic protection. I had a patient a few years ago, an African lady and her husband had business interests in this country so she was always coming and going, coming and going, coming and going. And she came, went, got home back to Africa once and her husband had taken all the photographs of her down. I know, that's a bit dodgy, isn't it? And he's obviously wanting to get rid of her and from that moment on she started to get sick and so she felt, "Well he's obviously put some sort of spell on me." So, I was treating her for high blood pressure and some just general stressy things and she had told me about this, I do like the way people tell herbalists all sorts of weird and strange things, don't you? It's because they think you're weird and strange. So, in a way it's good to have an image of being weird and strange, because then people will tell you things they wouldn't tell anybody else, which is often the key to their healing, isn't it? And she said, "Well, he must have put a spell on me somewhere and must have got the medicine man to put a spell and I can't find it. What am I going to do about it? Can you do anything for it?" And I thought, "Well, I don't want to get into battle with the medicine man, that's silly isn't it, always avoid psychic battles, not a good idea. So I gave her some Mugwort, I said "Hang the Mugwort over the bed", because it's a herbal protection which he won't know about and it worked really, really well actually. It worked well, for quite a long time it worked. She should have left him, of course, but she didn't leave him because their business interests were too twiddled out, entwined, and she should have really left him, let that go, but there you go.

Myrhh (*Commiphora molmol*)

I had a dream

I have a patient at the moment actually, who's got an ovarian cyst. She actually had two and one cleared up years ago after seeing a shaman in Brazil—did some sort of ceremony, and the other one has been there so long, it's not quite calcified, it's just a solid hard lump. It's not a real problem but it's a bit uncomfortable and she's worried— because her mother died of ovarian cancer—that it might be turning cancerous inside. So, she goes in and has blood tests or whatever every now and then to make sure. And she came round one day and I'd been trying to get rid of this without any success at all, shouldn't think like that should I? No. And she came in one day and said, "I had a dream", I said, "What did you dream about?" She said, "I dreamt about Myrrh, maybe it can help me." So, I gave her Myrrh and the cyst actually started going down. I haven't the faintest idea how or why Myrrh is helpful, I don't know, maybe I was thinking too scientifically, can't just be stimulating the immune system can it? No. I don't know, it's very odd isn't it, but it did start going down. Patients, like customers, of course, are always right. Do you ever get that thing where, because I like to have my herbs in the consulting room and they say, "Oh what's Lemon Balm used for?" and you say "Ah, you!" It's amazing, isn't it? Synchronicity, people get drawn to things. Anyway, back to the patient, last hospital visit was a couple of months ago and it had actually gone down. We will wait and see, won't we. And she said, she also said, she'd had it so long she hadn't noticed how discomforting it was. With it starting to go she noticed the whole pressure easing up and that was quite good because it made her think about pelvic energy flow and getting that unblocked, so she was starting to do some exercises to, which are also a benefit, of course. Keep the energy flowing there.

Nettle (Urtica dioica)

Phlegmatic superfluities

There is no doubt about the dryness of Nettles. Being a dry person myself, I find that excessive consumption of Nettles can dramatically dry out my system and I need to add Mallow[47] if I intend to take them for more than a day or two. As to heat, going to stroke the Nettles, I feel them to be moving rather than warming. The Martian quality that Culpeper mentions is more in the realm of activating rather than classically warming, but in the Galenic classification the closest we can get to that property is warming, so there they get placed. The good old usage of flogging ourselves with Nettles for stiffness due to cold and damp works

---

[47] Christopher may well have been referring to Marshmallow (*Althaea officinalis*) here, most likely the root, but also possibly Common Mallow (*Malva sylvestris*), Hollyhock (*Alcea rosea*) or any Tree Mallow (*Lavatera* spp.) that was to hand, according to bendle, who knows about these things. [Ed.]

because they banish damp and put some movement back into the joints. Have a read of Culpeper. A favourite quote is that Nettles "consume the phlegmatic superfluities in the body of man, that the coldness and moistness of Winter hath left behind."[48] Phlegmatic superfluities being diagnosed by heavy, stiff, dragging steps.

In love with them

I have lately been using Nettle root and Yarrow (fresh plant tinctures) for benign prostate hyperplasia and getting better results than I had with Saw Palmetto critical carbon dioxide extracts. Could just be because these are my local herbs and I am in love with them.

Only a veneer

My favourite story though is this, I was teaching basic humoral practice to a beginners' class. There was a young woman sitting at the back of the class and I could see she was notching up the points for herself as we discussed the phlegmatic type. I mentioned Nettle tea as a good constitutional remedy for phlegmatic people. The next week she came to the class and announced that she was leaving London and going back home to Australia. She told us that she had come to London some years ago intending to stay only a while and had got stuck here. One week of regular Nettle tea had cleared her excess phlegm and she was off back to a drier atmosphere. London is, of course, built on a marsh and the damp character of the city underlies it still. People might only see the air/fire rush and bustle of modern life but that is only a veneer.

All-time favourite

What a nice question to answer. It enables me to answer with my all-time favourite herbal medicine. My favourite preparation is dried wild Apricots and dried Nettles, with a little Bitter Orange peel (to help absorption), macerated in red wine. Dose is around one to four tablespoons daily. I make that just because I like it but I also keep a 1:1 fresh plant tincture which works well, in pregnant women for example.

---

[48] Culpeper, *Culpeper's Complete Herbal*, 179.

Passion Flower (Passiflora incarnata)
Simple joys

A short story. This starts with the diuretic index of a herb, which is the proportion of students who go out to pass water following blind tasting of a herb in class. Up until last month the best I had observed was Burdock root which had an index of 80%. Tasting several herbs over the course of a day on nervines with an experienced group of students had my first 100% index, including myself, with a totally unexpected herb—Passiflora. This was the first time I have used Passiflora in this context and a completely unexpected outcome. The other herbs that day had fairly expected outcomes, usually about ten or twenty per cent. Kava kava got eighty per cent but that was not unexpected. I have a patient with a benign but seriously swollen prostate, who wishes to avoid hospitals due to events in his medical history. I had been treating him for testicular cancer, with some success so he had faith that I could help him reduce his prostate and recover the simple joys of uninterrupted peeing once more. Although wishing to avoid hospitals, he is not beyond arranging tests. I had given him Saw Palmetto, with some small success and then added Nettle root and then Small-Flowered Willowherb (*Epilobium parviflorum*) with no improvement. He was on alpha blockers which had ceased to work, and I had made up a Lobelia cream as a substitute, again with no real improvement. So, I thought let's try the Nettle root again but with the addition of Passiflora. And it worked really well and has continued to work for a month so far. I told him the story about the diuretic index and why I gave him the Passiflora and he said that as a child he had been quite ill and his mother had given him a lot of Passiflora, for various reasons. So, this is a herb that obviously benefits him especially. Wonderful things herbs!

Pellitory of the Wall (Parietaria judaica)
Rearranging itself

Also, I treated a little boy this year with kidney stones, it's really interesting isn't it, mind you children are amazing. He's only three and he had kidney stones, kidney stones, kidney stones and he kept making them. Fortunately, at that time they hadn't moved much so hadn't had the pain but there was something very wrong with his calcium metabolism and the hospital were trying to sort out what was wrong with his calcium metabolism and they were thinking about giving him that stuff you give to post-menopausal ladies, whatever they call them, bisphosphonate thingies to make sure the calcium stays in the bone, because the calcium wasn't staying in the bone, which is a bit horrible. And his mother came to see me and we put him on Corn Silk and Pellitory of the Wall and he did actually pass one stone after that which was a bit painful for him but the number of stones is going down, which I expected anyway, but also his calcium metabolism is rearranging itself. Whether that's anything to do with Pellitory of the Wall and Corn Silk or not I do not know, but I'm quite pleased with that. I think it probably is, don't you? Probably pure magic. Yes.

Peony (Paeonia lactiflora)

Being a serious herbalist

Epilepsy, this will quickly remind you that you have to treat the person not the condition. We tend to get taken in by a diagnosis of a serious pathology and find ourselves resorting to pathological thinking. There is an American Herbalist who tried the traditional treatment of wearing a piece of Peony root around her neck. She had no fits whilst wearing it and, being a serious herbalist, she verified by challenge and rechallenge.

Peppermint (Mentha x piperita)

Four actions

The first impression is cooling—in the mouth and on the skin. Exhibiting my superior knowledge of pharmacology (or indeed, of toothpaste), I say that is because of the high evaporation rate of menthol. This cooling effect applies to any mint and may be used with profit by adding the herb, or essential oil, to light creams for hot, itchy skin—a trick which I first learned from Chinese formulae. The second impression is clearing of the sinuses and head. This action does not last. The third impression is of a cooling then warming action in the solar plexus area, followed by a relaxant/wind clearing action. Cue for some of the class to burp freely and loudly. The fourth action is a little sweatiness with warm hands and face. Cue for the introduction of the technical term "peripheral vasodilation"—which is a nicely poetic phrase. The warming action is more noticeable in longer use by general improvement of circulation in some people.

Plantain (*Plantago major, P. lanceolata*)

I'll try and track this down

I still collect Plantain seeds every year. I have a traditional recipe for ladies who've had miscarriages. And if you've had a miscarriage and you've been to the hospital and they say they don't know why you've had a miscarriage, just go away and try again, that's OK. But you're going to worry, aren't you? One of the lovely things about herbal medicine is that there is always something people can do, it's amazing, there's always something people can do. The folk tradition is you take seven Plantain seeds every day during the pregnancy and they stick the baby in the womb. At least I think it's a folk tradition. Last year I thought, well I'll try and track this down, and I looked through all my books and I couldn't find it anywhere, I'm beginning to suspect that I made it up.

The verticality of Plantains

What I love about Greater Plantain is how tough it is on the outside, and yet if you rub it, it's really soft inside. So perhaps if we pass the leaves round, have a rub, you'll see that it's really soft on the inside. I was told many years ago that I shouldn't talk about a herb without actually having it in my presence. Plantain is a herb that lies flat to the ground, the root is very short, just penetrating the top layer of the soil, its leaves spread out as if to protect the bare earth in which it often grows. The Saxon name is Waybroad—the broad-leafed herb that grows in the way in the path. Its whole being is horizontal, Greater Plantain especially, with hardly any vertical component. It's an interesting exercise, just thinking about this, I just thought we could do an exercise on verticality of herbs, couldn't we? We'd give them a vertical component factor, or a horizontal component factor. Dandelion's interesting isn't it, it's the opposite to Plantain, so in a way it connects to the earth in the air. But the Plantain doesn't. Greater Plantain (*Plantago major*), what it show us when we look at it, is it protects and heals surfaces. It protects the path from people walking on it. So, that's what it does, it protects and heals surfaces. The Ribwort Plantain (*Plantago lanceolata*) has quite a different look about it doesn't it? Ribwort is a much more vertical plant, it's much more orientated towards the air which shows that it's better for the lungs. But, it doesn't have that surface healing thing to such a degree as the Greater Plantain does. And that's indeed how people use it, isn't it? They tend to use Ribwort for lungs, though I quite often use a combination of the two.

Their energy is different. The chemistry is practically the same, but their energy is different. So *Plantago major*, the Greater Plantain, protects and heals surfaces outside and inside the body—in a way it's a healing herb *par excellence*. I'm a great weed man myself, are you a weed person?

Bloody brilliant

One of the Native American names of course for Waybroad, for Plantain, is Englishman's Foot, because when the English made paths across America, they obviously left the Plantain behind, so it obviously fell off their feet didn't it? I got told a story once by a Native American, he said there was a lady in his town who was a bit of a bother, she was always asking for things and this and that and the other, and what should I do for this and what should I do for that? And he bumped into her in the street one day and he was trying to be polite and get away, but she wouldn't, she wasn't that sort of person, she stood in front of him and said, "I want to get pregnant, what can I do?" And he said, "Plantain", after seeing it at his feet. Bloody brilliant, and it was, it worked.

Polypody of the Oak (*Polypodium vulgare*)

It sinks down

Pure melancholy is earth, so it sinks down in the body. So, a classic symptom for melancholic accumulation is constipation, basically. It's blockage in the lower half of the body. One of the main herbs for pure melancholy in the lower half of the body was Polypody of the Oak. It's a fern and it grows on trees and it runs right along the branch. If you're using it for melancholy always use the one that grows on Oak, because Oak is the most earthy and a heavier tree. It actually tastes of Liquorice and while one of the main symptomatic actions is just for constipation, it's for curing melancholy in the lower half of the body. Burnt, heavy dull pains, melancholy, blockages, obstructions.

Prickly Ash (*Zanthoxylum americanum, Z. clava-herculis*)

Must be your circulation

OK, Prickly Ash. Zanthoxylum, isn't that a nice word? Zanthoxylum. Those are serious looking trees aren't they, Prickly Ash trees? I always like to say, to beginner students, I take them round Chelsea Physic Gardens and I show them the Prickly Ash tree and I say, "What do you think that's for?" And I say, "That's for prickling people." They eat the berries and get that nice hot thing. I use Prickly Ash, I use it as an alterative, so I tend to use it more in cases of cancer, tumours, that sort of thing where there's circulatory problems as well. So I tend to think of it first as an alterative, but we do also think of it as a circulatory remedy. The thing I've noticed about Prickly Ash is it tends to work mostly on small arteries, it works more on getting the blood out than getting it back in again. So occasionally when I've used Prickly Ash in aches and pains in the legs, for example, they've got worse. Because more blood was coming into the legs. So now, I tend to use it with Yarrow for peripheral circulatory problems, the blood comes back again and doesn't just stay there causing problems.

We treated an elderly man a few years ago, he was getting up to eighty years old, he was still very fit, he was still working part time as a photographer and his favourite occupation was golf and he'd play golf two or three times a week. And he was getting aches and pains in his legs and I said, "Well, it's probably your circulation", he said "It can't be my circulation, I've been to hospital and they've done all the tests and they say it's not my circulation." If you're an elderly person, and you're getting aches and pains in your legs and there's nothing else wrong with you, you're basically fit, it must be your circulation. So, let's try Hawthorn, Prickly ash and Yarrow, let's do the whole thing. Move from the heart down through the arteries, back up through the veins. Hawthorn, Prickly Ash, Yarrow. Three months and he was fine, his aches and pains practically went. I treated him for about six months in all and the end of six months he was back playing golf and happy and he felt alive, so I gave him the recipe. Whether he's had to do it again or not I don't know. Because it's a bit silly for him to pay to come back and see me, "if it happens again, you can just go and buy the herbs from the shop, couldn't you?"

Raspberry Leaf (*Rubus ideaus*)

A soft furry blanket

I don't have a Raspberry leaf to hand, they don't grow in my garden. The soil isn't quite right. I've got a few Blackberries, brought over by the pigeons, no doubt. I think about Raspberry leaf as a soft, furry blanket. I think that much pins it down really. It's very soft to the touch and that softness of the touch actually gets inside the body and soothes and soothes. It's also, like most of the Rose family, toning. Think of the Rose family as gentle but firm astringents. So, it tones. Its toning action is concentrated on the lower body, on the lower abdomen around the womb and the pelvic area. Of course, it's the famous Romany remedy for facilitating birth. I generally advise people to take it only in the last three months, three cups of tea a day. It's a nice drinkable tea. Mainly because you get bored of it if you're taking it for longer. I think the last three months is good enough. You must take it for at least one month because it takes one month to build the tone into the womb and a toned womb feels strong and relaxed and well able to cope. Also, in the last couple of weeks or so I'd add either Motherwort tincture or sometimes two or three Cloves which can just be popped into the Raspberry leaf tea.

A bit grumbly in the tummy

My favourite remedy for colic, if I'm out in the wilds or somewhere like Hampstead Heath and getting a bit grumbly in the tummy because I'd rushed my tea at the lovely tea and scone place, is fresh Raspberry leaves. Just chew, just the baby ones from the end of the branch and just chew them. It's better with spasm to just chew gently and let the herb act slowly and slowly and slowly in the system. Same goes if, say, using Ginger in spasm. Just put it in hot water and sip, sip, sip. That's the way to do it. I have used Raspberry leaf tea for thrush in babies' mouths, just make the strong tea and spray. That works quite well. And King's[49] also says that probably one of the best sources is jam and they use Raspberry or Blackberry jam for children's colicky, upsetty, diarrhoeary things. I think, given that we love talking about flavonoids, jam is probably, logically, chemically a good way of taking flavonoids. It tastes nice, anyway. And finally, Raspberries themselves, the dried Raspberries, well the fresh Raspberries my teacher always used to make into vinegar, Raspberry vinegar, gargling for sore throats, which is good. The dried Raspberries, I got this tip from a Chinese herbalist, they're used for a weak bladder. In fact, if you carry the dried Raspberries around with you and just chew a few, you can go all the way from one place to the next without worrying about finding where the toilet is, no matter how weak your bladder is. You can buy the dried Raspberries in Chinese

---

[49] Felter and Lloyd, *King's American Dispensatory*, 1682. [Ed].

herb shops but they're not very nice, they're over dried. It's best to dry them yourself at home so pick a few now on your way home and dry them in a dehydrator or something like that, a nice thing to chew anyway. That's Raspberries.

Rhubarb (Rheum officinale, R. palmatum)

A nice young man as well

The best humoral balancer we have. Earth, air, fire and water should all stay in their place. If any element builds up it will overflow its place and finish up where it does not belong, leading to imbalance and illness. A good example: I treated a forty-year-old woman, an earth/fire lady, stuck in an emotionally abusive marriage (to an alcoholic) and with a responsible job. She was tired, not nourished on any level and in high-coping depression with not enough energy left to sort her life out. Given Rhubarb as a simple for three months she left her husband and found a new job at the other end of the country, and a nice young man as well.

Rose (Rosa spp.)

You could liberate them

I remember treating a patient of mine once, I treated her for a while, she was a fashion journalist. She said, "I don't think it's the most useful job in the known universe, is it?" It didn't satisfy her anyway. One of the things often with patients is that it is their jobs that are making them ill and you say to them that you're not going to get better until you change your job, basically. Change your job! Shall I give you a tip I got from a herbalist I know? If a patient wants to change their job or find new work but their job is tiring them out and they're too tired to change their job. Well, I use relaxing herbs, like Vervain and things like that are very good. But, when my friend was just starting on herbal medicine she got, well she thought she got a job in the Dominican Republic working for a charity with local healers but when she got there, they hadn't heard about her. So, she'd landed in a foreign country with hardly any money, nowhere to live and no work. So, she went down the market, as you do, and talked to the herbalists and one lady there said, "This is just between you and me, it's very important, make yourself a bath with yellow Rose petals and you pour it all over you and your life changes."

I've done this lots of times with patients now. It really works. It might be placebo effect, who knows. Who cares? Yellow Rose petals, don't buy them, you must pick them. Well, there's lots of yellow Roses around London, you could, as we said in the '60s, liberate them, couldn't you?

Rosebay Willowherb, Fireweed (*Epilobium angustifolium*)
Left to itself, it heals

Circumpolar, temperate to arctic ecologies. Rosebay was originally most common after forest fires. It heals the damaged earth, putting down deep tap roots to draw up minerals and sending out rhizomes to spread the goodness around.[50] It was rare in the UK until the railways came. It is now common beside motorways (the fluffy fruit helps its seeds to spread) and on damaged land everywhere. Left to itself it heals and then dies back, allowing other wildflowers to grow back. The best advice for new nature reserves is just to let it be for a couple of years. The pith is sweet with a mild spicy aftertaste. It is eaten raw or fermented. It can be used to make beer. Native Americans make jellies and syrups. Siberian shaman say that it protects against the toxic effects of Fly Agaric[51]—mainly gastrointestinal overactivity including spasm. It is also used for irritable bowel and candida, as a tea. It works well. If you are picking it for tea do not pick in flower as it fertilises itself and then spreads fluff all over the kitchen floor.

Rosemary (*Salvia rosmarinus* syn. *Rosmarinus officinalis*)
From the heart outwards

My main restorative herb for the circulation is Rosemary. Who likes Rosemary? Lots of people like Rosemary, I see. If you take Rosemary, you feel that it acts from the heart outwards. Things like Ginger and Capsicum do to some extent, but a lot of warming herbs don't really

---

[50] Suitably, given one of its names (it readily springs up after ground has been cleared by fire), Fireweed was the first plant to colonise London's bombsites of the second world war. [Ed.]

[51] A favourite source of Christopher's, Maud Grieve, notes that in Kamchatka, Siberia, ale made from Fireweed is combined with Fly Agaric, noting that this makes the ale "still more intoxicating." See: Grieve, *A Modern Herbal*, 848. Wasson points out that in Siberia, Fly Agaric was taken with Fireweed. See: Robert Gordon Wasson, *Soma: Divine Mushroom of Immortality* (Harcourt Brace Jovanovich, 1968), 152, 186. [Ed.]

do that, they don't really get deep into the heart and then act out, but Rosemary acts from the heart. In Germany, you can actually get in the chemist a Rosemary cream for rubbing in over the heart. Isn't that a nice idea? When I found that out I immediately made Rosemary cream for rubbing over the heart, for physical or for emotional things. If you make a cream for rubbing over an emotionally bruised area, that's obviously going to be beneficial, isn't it? If you make a cream for rubbing over a physically damaged area it's also going to be beneficial because, what tends to happen is when we're ill in any particular part of the body or any particular part of the body isn't working, we ignore it. We say, "Well, if I ignore it, maybe it'll get better." But that's not the case, of course, is it? So, a lot of the time we make creams for rubbing in. I like just a nice little bit of Rosemary ointment, something like that, couple of drops of essential oil to perk it up and rub that in. It's very nice. Very often when we get elderly people coming in with all sorts of pains and complaints and things and often everything arises just purely from poor circulation, just purely from cold and a herb like Rosemary taken over two or three months will banish everything and I've seen really severe arthritis banished just by taking Rosemary and that's not going to happen with everybody obviously, most people are going to have to have other things as well, but I have seen that, when the problems are just down to circulation, just down to cold.

The Queen of Hungary and the Prince of Poland

There's a nice story about Rosemary water, I can't remember her name now, the Queen of Hungary rather fancied the Prince of Poland. I suppose if you're a Queen you haven't got much choice have you, really? Looked around, she said, "Well, the only half-decent man around here is the Prince of Poland, a good few years younger than me so before I go and see him, I'd like to look a bit younger." And she had a court herbalist and the court herbalist made up a magic elixir for her to look younger and it was basically just distilled Rosemary. Just Rosemary water. And apparently it worked really well. She bathed in it and washed her hair in it and things like that. If your circulation is slowing down, your skin tends to lose its shininess, doesn't it? So, you use circulatory remedies to get the shine and the tone and the vigour and the youthfulness back into the skin. And apparently, you can still buy Hungarian Rosemary water in Hungary. In fact, I had a patient come back a few years ago, he was losing his hair and he'd been on holiday to Hungary and he bought this bottle of stuff to rub into his hair and it was about, I don't know, fifty pounds or something for a little bottle like that and I opened it and smelt it and all I could smell was Rosemary. I said, "Well, I'm sure it will work, yes I'm sure it will work." Especially since he paid that much for it.

Continuities

And people would in the old days, they'd give sprigs of Rosemary, if you were going away, so that shows that you would always remember me. So, it's a symbol, of friendship, it's a symbol of remembrance. I think it's nice that it's a symbol, it also actually physically strengthens the memory by improving the blood flow to the brain. I always say to people when they ask me about magical herbal medicine that if the magical uses proposed in a particular book or whatever, if they're congruent with the actual physical uses of the herb, then the person probably knows what they're talking about, you see what I mean? There must be a continuity like that, the magic and the spiritual uses must be congruent with the physical uses, because there's a continuity between the body and the spirit. And if there isn't any congruence with what you know about the herb then, don't do it basically. It doesn't mean anything. That's Rosemary.

Sage (*Salvia officinalis*)

Holds energy in the centre

Here's a Sage leaf from my garden. I love the delicate wrinkly pattern on the leaf. It shows its holding quality. They do say of Sage that if it's growing strong in the garden then the woman is in charge of the house. You might like to know that. It's a favourite offering of the Ancient Greeks to the Gods. They'd burn it on the alter and it would go up and please the Gods, bring them down with a smile on their face to help you. When you've tasted it, I hope anyway, you feel the way it draws into the centre, it draws the vitality, the vital heat, your energy of life into the centre of the body and holds it there. This is how it works with hot flushes and night sweats, either by biochemistry or by innate virtues. The "stops sweating" action is notable and reliable. It's very good for scattered states. I use it a lot for, after infections, when everything's been scattered and everything needs to be brought back to the centre again.

Holding the centre and preventing dispersal seems to be the main activity of Sage, an activity that is carried over to the central nervous system and is particularly useful in elders, debilitated people, people who are too easily scattered, including in psychosis, and for grief, especially at the loss of a child. The acetylcholine-sparing effect explains its traditional use to help focus, sensory enhancement, concentration, good quality sleep and memory. It is my herb of choice for poor memory from anxiety, which is down to lack of focus. The Grete Herball[52] recommends it for epilepsy.

Nice combination

I know herbalists that are working on a combination of Wood Betony and Sage for early Alzheimer's and saying that they're getting some results. I don't know, it's worth a try. You can't go far wrong with that. Nice combination. The idea about using Betony is to make sure, because Betony is a head herb, it appropriates to the head. So, make sure that most of the remedy gets up to the head and isn't wasted where it's not needed.

Empty heat

One of those expressions I picked up in Chinese medicine is "empty heat". It's a nice expression, I think it informs us quite well, empty heat—they're sweating and having heat symptoms but you can't treat them by cooling them down because there is no internal heat. So, you use a warm remedy like Sage, a warm, dry remedy like Sage. And Sage is wonderful as an adjunct in treating people with HIV. It's a superb herb because it'll stop night sweats just like that, within a few days. A good cup of cold Sage tea with a bit of honey in, taken before you go to bed. It'll usually stop the night sweats within a few days.

---

[52] The Grete Herball, a compendium of medicinal plant knowledge, notes that "The wyne that sawge is soden in is good for them ye haue the fallynge euyll." *The Grete Herball* (London: Peter Treveris, 1526), https://quod.lib.umich.edu/e/eebo2/A03048.0001.001/1:21?rgn=div1;view=toc. Search contents for: De Saluia. Sawge. Ca. CCC. Vi. Thanks to Frances Watkins, herbalist, historian, educator and friend of Christopher's, for pointing me to this source. Also, John Gerard, writing 71 years later, argues that Sage "taketh away shaking, or trembling of the members." *John Gerard, The Herball or Generall Historie of Plantes* (London: John Norton, 1597), 624. http://www.biolib.de/gerarde/gerarde_herball.pdf. And Culpeper, writing in 1653, states that Sage "helps the falling-sickness". Culpeper, *Culpeper's Complete Herbal*, 28. [Ed.]

Just think about the patient

The only time that Sage doesn't work particularly well in menopausal complaints is when the woman is hot, of a hot constitution. So basically, fiery women, because Sage is a bit warm in itself and doesn't actually help that. So, then I add in something cooling. We used to add in Motherwort which lowers thyroid activity—it's used for hyperthyroid, overactive thyroid. Therefore, it lowers the metabolic rate a little bit and if we give Sage and Motherwort then that will clear up 90%, 95% of all hot flushes. The rest you have to, well the other 5% is the same with anything in herbal medicine. When you make general formulas which cover most people, there's always some people it won't cover. You have a formula which works on a particular set of symptoms and it always works and then one day it doesn't work. And the best way around that is to stop thinking about the symptoms, which is what you should've been doing all along of course, and just think about the patient.

Sage helps deal with that

I like to use Sage for women that have had miscarriages or whose baby was stillborn because it dries up the milk that might have been, because it dries up the milk very quickly. It re-establishes a hormonal balance very quickly and it helps with the grief, with the emotional aspects as well as the physical aspects. I suppose grief and sadness is something that comes more to us as we're getting older. It's always a bit sad isn't it, when you have older patients and I say, "Shall I call you by your Christian name or your second name, which would you prefer?" And some people say, "No one's called me by my Christian name for about ten years, because all my friends have died." It's always a bit sad, isn't it? So, there's a lot of grief around, Sage helps deal with that.

By degrees

In the old herbals, if you look in the old Galenical system, Sage is said to be hot in the first degree and dry in the second degree. There's three degrees of hotness and dryness. So hot in the first degree means warm. As we know from Sage, it's a warming herb but it's not really hot or burning. Dry in the second degree means it's really quite seriously dry. It's a very drying herb. It's a bit astringent to taste. But to taste it's not as astringent as you would think that would give it two degrees of dryness.

Just a little bit astringent. In actual fact, the general properties of Sage are very drying throughout the system. They dry up secretions so that's why it's given that extra degree of dryness.

Chew

I remember doing a workshop once down in a garden in the countryside and there was a woman there, her mouth was full of mouth ulcers for, I don't know, for whatever reason. And I said, "Oh, you need Sage." She said, "I've been drinking Sage, I've been drinking Sage. It hasn't made any difference at all." I said, "Eat some, just chew some. Just pick a couple, there's a nice Sage bush here, coincidentally. Just pick a couple of leaves and chew them." Fifteen minutes and all the ulcers had gone, just chewing the Sage. So, the traditional way of taking Sage wasn't actually to take a Sage tea, the traditional way of taking Sage was to eat the Sage. In Surrey, which is now suburbs, but used to be deepest countryside, they say if you eat five leaves of Sage every morning at breakfast you live for a very long time. They used to make Sage sandwiches.

Sage total capacity point

I don't think I could drink it every day even if I think I could live to be one hundred and fifty. After a couple of weeks of drinking Sage, I reach a Sage total capacity point, where every single cell in my body has got its hit of Sage essential oil, there's just not any room for anymore. Some people can drink it forever but I have a cut-off point. So, let's just say it's a herb with a strong personality. It's a herb, which, although it can be used for men and women, is a friendly herb for women. I have a picture of Sage—I tend to make pictures of the herbs that I use the most. Just a little thumbnail sketch of the herb and that picture of Sage is of an earth mother. I think of a woman in the farmyard, a good solid looking woman. And she's standing in the farmyard and she's doing what farm wives do. She's feeding the hens, and she's feeding the pigs and she's feeding the children, and a lot of the children aren't hers. Because she's such a nice motherly type, they're from all around the place. And she's feeding them and nourishing them but she won't let you get away with anything. You have to behave yourself. That's Sage for you, very nourishing but with a strong personality and a direct opinion of how things should be done. Sage informs your body of how things should be done. That's what it does, by taking it on a regular basis if that's the herb that suits you, that's how it works. It just keeps your body on the track and therefore keeps you healthy well into old age.

Leaf between leaves

Another reason why Sage is good as we get older is because it helps the memory. It says in the old herb books that if you put a leaf of Sage in a book, one leaf of Sage between two leaves of a book, you remember what's written on the pages of that book. But you have to read them first. That's how you can always tell a herbal student. If you go into their house, you take a book off the shelf, Sage leaves fall out all over the place. So, there we are, there's a tip for you. Need a big bush I expect.

A reasonable strategy

I've also used it three times, four times actually, for prolactin-secreting tumours of the pituitary gland. I use the tincture, equal parts Sage and Thuja and then back that up with a couple of cups of Sage tea to really get the Sage in there just to bring the prolactin levels down. It works very, very well. I had three women, out of the four, three women got pregnant, which is the main reason, of course, why women came to see me with prolactin secreting tumours. And one woman actually had two babies each time, might be the Sage doing it and bringing the prolactin down again. It's a reasonable strategy. The orthodox strategy for prolactin-secreting tumours is to give the drug for a couple of years and cross your fingers because very often the whole thing will just go away then you don't have to do the operation, which is very tricky. So, doing the same thing with the Sage and Thuja is a reasonable strategy. Just measure prolactin levels and see how you're going and see if you're having success.

And she did

I also use it for cystic breasts, painful lumpy breasts before the period. I had a lady a few years ago, had very painful lumpy breasts before her periods and that cleared up really nicely with Sage and then she moved away and rang me up and said she'd got pregnant, and I thought, well, she shouldn't be using Sage. It doesn't really matter because when you're pregnant everything changes and hopefully her cystic breasts would go away but they didn't. Her breasts were still really painful for the pregnancy. So, in the end, because she'd actually got pregnant using the Sage, I thought, well, why not use the Sage and she did and she was happy and she had a baby.

Really strong, good smelling Sage

One of my patients married a Turkish man and he went back to his grandmother's village in Turkey a couple of years ago. This was a two-day bus drive up into the mountains, and they got up into the mountains and they got to the village, there wasn't anybody there. Not a soul in the village, just the dogs and the chickens and tomatoes and things. No people, though. None whatsoever, they'd all gone. And they thought, what's happened here? All they can do is sit down and wait, so they sat down and waited. They waited quite a long time and at dusk the whole village came down out of the mountains with big sacks. And they asked, "Oh, what have you been doing?" And they said, "We've been gathering Sage, we've been gathering wild Sage from the mountains. It's Mayday, it's the day for gathering wild Sage." And they had these big sacks of wonderful smelling Sage. And my friend, because she's interested in herbs, she's a friend as well as a patient. Anyway, she said, "Oh, I'm interested in herbs and that's very nice Sage. Really strong, good smelling Sage. I'll go out tomorrow and gather some." And they said, "No you can't do that. The day is gone, I'm sorry. This is the only time of the year for gathering Sage, you mustn't gather it at any other time." Good! I like that, it's nice to hear that the stories are still going, things are still going.

I'll let you know

I gave Sage to a patient recently to smudge her house, and she said, as soon as she started burning it, the dogs started howling and the children started screaming. So obviously she's upset the spirit of the house and the Sage is a bit pushy. So, then I said the thing to do then is to go round and put salt in all the corners. Because you want to soak up the energy rather than try and push it out because it's going to push back. I don't know what happened yet, hopefully it worked, I'll let you know.

St John's Wort (*Hypericum perforatum*)

With consistently good results

I have used high doses of St John's wort, 10 ml three times daily of a good tincture, to help people reduce their morphine dose, with consistently good results. All of these people were dying and I was taught that St John's wort worked best on pain in people near death.

Feet firmly on the ground

I once gave St John's wort tea to an adult education class in a blind tasting. I have done this before and comments have included tingly ears, comforting, soothing, cleansing, enters the heart chakra, rich, warm and pleasant. This time it obviously had a very bad effect on one of the class. She went very quiet but wouldn't discuss her reaction. We gave her some Vervain tea and Rosemary to smell—as first aid, but she stayed quiet and rushed out at the end of the class. I phoned her the next day but there was no answer. Being quite worried, I kept trying. I spoke to her on the second day and she said that she had been extremely depressed and suicidal and had not slept at all due to visitations from dark things in the night. The tea had revealed old feelings, which she had thought she had buried. Fortunately, she knew how to deal with the feelings. She remarked that they were different from previous feelings in that, although they were just as intense, she felt her feet firmly on the ground the whole time. By this time, she was feeling much better. She mentioned that she had taken St John's wort tincture before with no bad effects so I suggested she take a few drops, put some Mugwort over her bed and she would be fine, and she was.

Comments from the rest of the class included drying inside the head, too heady, relaxing, sedative, warming, relaxed body and alert mind. 80% thought it was mood altering and 20% not so, the most interesting comment was, "allows me to fill my skin" and one person said, "doesn't allow me to pretend to myself."

I myself, felt quite disorientated, sad and cut off from the spirit and had to take a long walk to regain myself, but maybe I was just picking up on the student's feelings. When I got home, Non remarked that taking the herb in a basement at night was probably not helpful since it is a herb that is best taken in the sunshine. I write this as John Denver sings "Sunshine almost always makes me high."

Omelettes and amulets

I had just been to see a patient with chronic fatigue syndrome who had taken St John's wort tea for shingles and had been extremely giggly for three days. I was always taught never to give the herb for severe depression. In our folk tradition, stepping on St John's wort before bed means that the fairies will pick you up and carry you around all night—sufficient reason for avoiding the herb in psychotic depression I suppose. The Grete Herbal[53] recommends the herb as a diuretic and, with eggs, for jaundice. St John's wort omelette. It has been used since ancient times to drive out demons, but as an amulet.

You turn round and it disappears

Have you done dreaming with St John's wort? You know people talk about power plants, the shamans talk about power plants and Ayahuasca and Belladonna and stuff like that. St John's wort is a power plant, with no equal I think really. So, what St John's wort does, of course, is it facilitates lucid dreaming, which is where you wake up in the dream, you're aware of the dream, you can then govern and direct the dream. I quite often use dreaming strategies with patients if it's appropriate and that's one good one. Especially if people are lost in their dreams. You know the old thing that you told your children, "I was dreaming I was being followed by a monster, I was very, very scared" and you say, "Well, what you do is you stop and you turn round and it disappears." Well, no one's been taught that in this society, but if you tell patients with huge confidence they can do it then they can do it and they will do it. And either use St John's wort or Mugwort.

A wort for St John

So, I always think St John's wort is for people who are suffering from an attack of the St John's. St John, of course, is St John the Baptist and what did St John the Baptist do? He went out in the desert and dressed in skins and ate locusts and generally flagellated himself, didn't he?

---

[53] *The Grete Herball*, 1526. https://quod.lib.umich.edu/e/eebo2/A03048.0001.001/1:21?rgn=div1;view=toc.
Search contents page for: De Iperyco. Herbe Iohñ/or saynt Io|hannis worte. Ca. CC.xix. [Ed.]

So, if at any stage in your life you find yourself in the middle of the desert, dressed in skins eating locusts, you know what herb to take. Now, that actually represents quite a nice picture of some of the usefulness of St John's wort, doesn't it?

Skullcap (*Scutellaria lateriflora, S. galericulata*)
Single most useful herb in psychosis

We always used *Scutellaria galericulata* when we had the market stall, many years ago. It is our local species. I got out of the habit when people started growing *S. lateriflora*, which seems more tolerant of a wider range of conditions—i.e., it is easier to grow. Also *S. galericulata* always grows in damp conditions, such as riverbanks where it can be difficult to pick. I strongly agree that Skullcap, of either species, is the single most useful herb in psychosis, whether or not people are taking the drugs. Indeed, I think that this is such a useful application that everyone should be out spreading the word. It dampens down the background anxiety level, making life more tolerable. The bitterness of *S. galericulata* also makes it a useful cooling herb, which was its main indication in the old herbals.

Valerian (*Valeriana officinalis*)
A nineteenth century French cavalry officer

Valerian is very, very good for airy people. Airy people always need calming and unknotting and soothing and spreading out. Had an interesting experience of Valerian a few years ago, I was doing a weekend workshop and we were drawing the plants in the herb garden, and the lady who was drawing Valerian pointed out how very erect, it's very straight, isn't it? Erect and beautiful, it's got this nice pink fluff that, she said it looks like a nineteenth century French cavalry officer. It really does. So, the reason why fiery people don't get on with Valerian, of course, is because the Cavalry officer will be telling them what to do and they don't want to do it. The airy person likes being told what to do, so they will do it.

It will revolt

I think we have all seen it misdiagnosed for insomnia. It's one of the first mistakes that beginning herbalists make. Still, mistakes exist for our learning. The classic insomnia due to fire is overexcitement.

So, the really classic insomnia due to fire is children on Christmas Eve. They're not worrying, are they? They're not thinking, "Oh my God, Santa Claus is going to come and eat me." They're just excited. Patients will come in and say they've got insomnia and you ask them if they can't sleep because they're worried or because their mind's full, especially when you start a new job or a project that you're getting excited about, and it's keeping them awake. And in those circumstances, you cannot use Valerian, because Valerian is not suitable for overexcitement. It won't respond to it. It will revolt against it. So, the main thing about Valerian is if there is a degree of anxiety, then Valerian is always useful. I use Valerian as a simple for acute anxiety. My preference is a fresh plant tincture of one- or two-year-old roots, garden grown.

Vervain (*Verbena officinalis*)

The noise level goes up

In Physiomedical terms, relaxant applies to a herb that loosens tension in tissue. The term does not relate to the modern use of the word relaxing—except in so far as the nervous system is itself a tissue. As a guiding principle, I consider a herb to be relaxing if I feel a relaxing effect on my bodily tension. Taken in a class, herbs such as Vervain are noticeably relaxing and stimulating—the noise level in the class goes up.

Letting go

In my journey so far, I see Vervain as a letting go herb based on relaxation of the upper body. This accounts for its use in asthma, as an emetic, for clearing the liver, as a diaphoretic, depression and exhaustion for people carrying too much or still carrying an illness after it should have been let go, people who think they can push through by willpower alone, workaholics and for promoting deep, healing sleep. Its indications overlap considerably with those of its flower remedy. If you give it as a simple your patient's lives often undergo a profound change. It is the only herb found in lists of both Saxon and Druidic sacred herbs. Despite the fact that they both came to live in the same country, they obviously occupied different head spaces but still both stood in need of letting go on a psychic level.

Might not finish the cup

Vervain is emetic at high doses, dose depending on the person. In many years of blind tasting of Vervain tea in classes we average around fifteen per cent strong feelings of nausea—enough for those people not to finish the cup. I always make fairly weak teas since this is the only way to appreciate all the flavours. My theory is that nauseating herbs work by over-relaxing the stomach.

Wormwood (*Artemisia absinthium*)

Charming, not

Charming is *not* a compliment—it means to put charms on people. Glamorous is not a compliment—glamour is tricking the eyesight. The first time I used the herb this way was for a student who had had a holiday romance. She knew in her heart that it had no future but her head kept dwelling on him. Wormwood tincture 5 ml three times daily banished him from her mind in three days. I have also used it in much smaller doses. For example, I had a patient who was wanting to move to a smaller house. Her husband was charmed by a lady estate agent who offered completely unsuitable properties. My patient preferred another agent who gave more sensible advice. I suggested Wormwood to break the spell but there was no way that he could be persuaded to take herbs. My patient thought that she could add a few drops to his wine. She tried this and it worked. It is beyond me how he didn't taste the Wormwood.

Here's something to do at weekend workshops. Make a love medicine from Rose petals following Culpeper's method of grinding them up in a pestle with granulated sugar. Keep adding Rose until you have a thick paste, roll this into balls and allow to dry overnight. Wrap the balls in a single Rose petal and then in foil. Take them home and give one or two to someone you fancy—but be careful who you choose! If you choose the wrong person the easiest way to get them to take Wormwood is to visit a trendy wine bar serving absinthe.

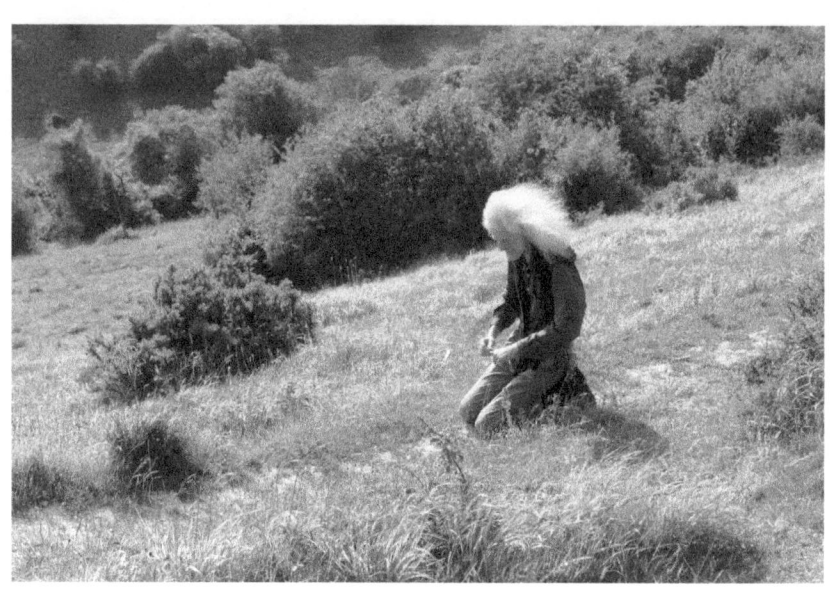

Photo by Vanessa Green

Seeds—Living Plants and Philosophy of Practice for Plant Medicine

My favourite bit

I'll tell you my story, shall I? When I was a child, we were brought up in a typical suburban house, typical suburban garden with a lawn and a vegetable patch and a bit at the end which was always my favourite bit, you know the bit at the end of the garden? It was particularly exciting in those days because we had an air raid shelter, with also a bonfire place and weeds. And I think there's a stage in your life, round about five or six years old, when you begin to realise that the world outside the family is composed of discreet objects—it isn't just a general blur of life outside the family. And I was about five, and I would sit at the end of the garden and I suddenly noticed the Red Deadnettle, I think that was the first individual plant that I noticed. I think that, at that moment the fairies planted the seed in my soul, maybe they did it earlier, I don't know, but that's the moment I remember.

It's wonderful

I remember saying to David Winston, the American herbalist, once, that we'd lost our ceremonies in this society, our rituals and our ceremonies. He said, "When you're picking plants don't you do it in a ceremonial manner?" I went, "Oh yeah!" Picking plants with a small group of herbalists is the most brilliant ceremony in the entire universe, it's better than going to church, it's wonderful.

It's a good exercise

Tell me, what's the first duty of a herbalist? What do you need to look after if the plants are going to be healthy. You need to look after the earth, don't you? The first duty of the herbalist is in regard to the earth, and nobody does that these days, do they? There's a general neglect of the earth, but if the earth isn't good then you can't grow strong healing plants. I always say to students it's only herbalists that can save the world. And you save the world by educating the people around you, your patients, and bringing back a love of nature and a respect for the earth herself. Holding hands, you hold hands with things. All those organisms that hold hands with each other in the earth, and all the plants holding their hands together. All the beings within an ecosystem hold hands, just as the herbs in an effective prescription hold hands. One exercise I do sometimes, if I'm not sure about the prescription is to imagine the herbs walking down the street holding hands, are they getting on with each other, or are they going, "Urgh!"? Right OK, I'll leave that one out, then. It's a good exercise, I think. And we as herbalists, we hold hands with our community and with the healing plants we use. I think Culpeper's dictum of "English Herbs for English Bodies"[1] is truest for the herbalist themselves rather than for their patients. You need to make a relationship with the herbs in your ecosystem and build on that relationship.

Spending time

Herbalists will heal the world. Because herbalists know about people and also about plants. So, they act as a bridge to reconnect people with nature. Herbalists are the nicest people on the planet, you know. I'd rather spend time with herbalists than with anyone else at all.

---

[1] Culpeper included this statement as a subtitle to The English Physician Enlarged— "*containing a complete a Method of Physic, whereby a Man may preserve his Body in Health; or cure himself, being Sick, for Three-pence Charge, with such Things only as grow in England, they being most fit for English Bodies."*
See: Nicholas Culpeper, *The English Physician Enlarged: With Three Hundred and Sixty Nine Medicines, Made of English Herbs, That Were Not in Any Impression until This*. (London: W. Baynes, 1799), https://wellcomecollection.org/works/tazb4r8a/items. [Ed.]

You can actually make it up

I have a general theory that if you're an established herbalist and you've been around the plants for a long time, you can actually make it up. It seems to be that if you develop a relationship with the plant, you can ask it to partake in new things for you to do, the plant must obviously be somewhat inclined in that direction anyway, and you can ask it to do new things for you.

Three inches off the ground

Mugwort, of course, is traditional, you stick it in your shoes when you're tired. Puts me in mind of a long pilgrimage I took down to Aylesbury for midsummer a few years ago. And I was walking, and after about two or three miles, I started to get blisters, I don't normally get blisters. And I thought, "That's all right, I'm a herbalist, I know what to do." I was stuffing Plantains in my socks. So, I sat down, stuffed some Plantain in my sock, didn't work. And I thought, "That's all right, I'm a herbalist, I know what to do". I should stuff some Dock leaves in my sock. I sat down, stuck some Dock leaves in my sock, didn't work. And Mugwort and then just about every single healing herb, I finished up about three inches above the ground. And it didn't work at all, but I suppose really, if you're going on a pilgrimage, you have to have a bit of suffering, don't you?

Always

There is always something that you can do.

Totally possible

I tend to think that the final examinations at herb schools should include a session where the students sit down somewhere and are then asked to heal everybody that walks past with just what they can see around them. It is totally possible, it is totally possible.

Donuts

We're reminded that people are basically donuts. Yes, your digestive tract is on the outside, the hole through the middle of the donut, it's not on your inside, it's on the outside. So, the same herbs that can be used for healing wounds on the skin can be used for healing wounds in the digestive tract. The only problem being that it's difficult to put a Plantain poultice on your stomach, so you have to drink the lot.

Tradition and direct knowing

The level of sophistication in traditional European medicine was, and is, profound. Look at the works of the Salerno school[2] and cast an eye over the Seven Books of Paulus Aegineta[3], as translated and published in the 19th century. My main teacher thought of herself as in the Physiomedical tradition. Check out Priest and Priest[4] for an elegant exposition of that tradition. It is clear to me that the basic principles in which all traditional medicines are rooted are demonstrated in the Physiomedical writings as much as in any other medical writings. Take as good a grasp of the basic principles and you can soar, within personal limitations, to the highest levels of sophistication. Inherited traditions are not the be all and end all of anything. Tradition is nothing unless it can change and flow with the times and it seems to me that Western herbal medicine is flowing and changing in the most exciting and exacting ways. Perhaps this makes it look like a "hodgepodge of various beliefs and practices" to an outsider. In the end there is no such thing as lost knowledge. The plants and our bodies know what they know. Direct knowing is much more useful in healing than any handed down tradition.

---

[2] Readers may be interested in the following two sources: Sha Ha, "A Review on Medicine in Medieval Times and the Multicultural Origin and Development of the Salerno Medical School," *Medicina Historica* 6, no. 2 (2022): e2022021, https://www.mattioli1885journals.com/index.php/MedHistor/article/view/11319/10937.
Violet Moller, *Map of Knowledge : How Classical Ideas Were Lost and Found—a History of Seven Cities* (London: Picador, 2020). [Ed.]

[3] Aegineta Paulus, *The Seven Books of Paulus Ægineta*, trans. Francis Adams (Sydenham: Sydenham Society, 1884), https://www.gutenberg.org/ebooks/author/55793. [Ed.]

[4] Priest and Priest, *Herbal Medication*. Also see these papers, available from the National Institute of Medical Herbalists (www.nimh.org.uk):
A.W. Priest, *Studies in Physiomedicalism. Paper 1. Historical and Philosophical.* (A.W. Priest, 1959).
A.W. Priest, *Studies in Physiomedicalism. Paper 2. Principles of Diagnosis.* (A.W. Priest, 1959).
A.W. Priest, *Studies in Physiomedicalism. Paper 3. Principles of Medication.* (A.W. Priest, 1961).
A.W. Priest, *Studies in Physiomedicalism. Paper 4. Materia Medica.* (A.W. Priest, 1962).
A.W. Priest, *Studies in Physiomedicalism. Paper 5. Principles of Therapeutics.* (A.W. Priest, 1963). [Ed.]

Feel better

Marigold is my desert island herb! If I get depressed on my island I will gaze at the flowers and feel better.

Three names

I think that plants, like T S Eliot's "Old Possum's Book of Practical Cats", have three names. A fancy Latin name for classification and introductions on formal occasions. A common English name for everyday usage, and a "deep and inscrutable singular name", which only it knows.

Humans name everything they can. It is a first question, "What's this called?" In Genesis 2:18, after God created the wild beasts and flying creatures, he presented them to Adam to name. "Whatever the man would call it, each living soul, that was its name." So, everything came forward to receive it's nomen: elephants, mice, snakes and cockroaches. Adam, first man and nominator—taming the beast, organising the delineations of chaos with words. Assigning a name is a magical act. It moves an object from the randomness of the fearful unknown into the communicable sphere of human experience. It becomes known. It may slide and slither, but once netted and named an object is caught. A name implies some understanding and bestows a "knowing" power over the object. It can be called by its name. Thus, the fear and superstition of divulging a personal name to a stranger. There are many folk tales and fairy stories on this theme, the most famous being Rumpelstiltskin. What is in a name? "A Rose by any other name would smell as sweet." But would it? A true name has a unique harmonic, a weft, running through the sound fabric of the word. To have the sort of power that mediaeval alchemists dreamt of, it would be necessary to know all the names of a herb, including the plant's private name. A secret it is wisely reluctant to yield.

Why do you ask?

Which reminds me of another eye-opening experience I had when I was a student. My teacher was treating an elderly West Indian man for high blood pressure, probably due to living in England, in the broadest sense. His wife would sit in the waiting room and chat to me as I dispensed and washed up. One day she came in with a bunch of Black Horehound (*Ballota nigra*) and asked me what it was. I was pleased to be able to give the herb a name and launched into a dissertation on its properties and uses, somewhat overanxious to demonstrate my new knowledge. She waited until I had run out of steam and then gave me a quizzical look. So, I said what I should have said first, "Why do you ask?" She replied that her spirits had come to her in the night and told her to go into the garden, pick this herb and rub it into her head.

You're my best friend

My favourite herb? Herbs are like friends, aren't they. They should be like friends, and at certain times of your life you've stronger relationships with certain friends, other times with other friends. You make friends with the herbs, so it's like asking who's your favourite friend, isn't it? You're my best friend.

Canadian Fleabane on a busy road

A few years ago, I carried out a simple exercise with the students, a space came up in the training clinic, they often do, and I thought to fill it with a bit of practical learning. We went outside and, oh there it is, Canadian Fleabane. Canadian Fleabane is the commonest large herb in central London, hardly anybody knows it's there, and nobody knows what it's used for. Do you know Canadian Fleabane? It's one of those plants that has a really hot taste too, an unexpectedly hot taste. Anyway, I said, "Go outside" to about a dozen students, "Find the Canadian Fleabane, it's growing round a tree on a busy road, ask it out loud." They were very brave, considering they were BSc students. I asked them to ask it out loud, "What are you used for?" and then sit with it for a bit, and then write down, and then we'll go in and we'll look it up. Every single thing they came up with was in the books. So, what do we use Canadian Fleabane for? It's used for warts on application, it's used as a diuretic, it's used for kidney stones, the French still use it apparently for rheumatism. Is that true? Any French people here? For throat inflammations and for internal bleeding. There's a very famous Eclectic recipe for internal bleeding, for stopping internal bleeding, which is Canadian Fleabane and Cinnamon essential oil. It's supposed to be the thing to stop internal bleeding[5]. The Native American use for Canadian fleabane was to breathe up the juice, just the smell of it, for sinusitis. It's got quite a sharp smell. And there it is.

---

[5] Please see: Felter and Lloyd, *King's American Dispensatory*, 726–727; and Ellingwood, *American Materia Medica*, 351–353. It is listed under *Erigeron* (*Erigeron canadensis* syn. *Conyza canadensis*). [Ed.]

Choosing herbs

Years and years and years ago, when the Wellcome Institute was still quite a nice place for alternative people, they had a Tibetan doctor come and I thought, well I shall go and listen to the Tibetan doctor because I was very interested in humoral medicine. It started off with Culpeper because that was one of the first books I had but that's very much his take on things. I loved the poetry in Culpeper and wanted to try and get into the poetry. So, I went to listen to the Tibetan doctor. At the end he said, "Any questions?" At the time, being a baby herbalist and only knee-high to a giraffe, the thing that worried me most, because what you're taught in university or college is that herbs have actions, which of course is a complete and total lie. Herbs do not have actions at all. Herbs have interactions. They interact with people. But you are taught actions so you get a whole list of diuretics and you think, what diuretic shall I give this patient, what diuretic, you don't know, no one tells you what to do. Well, no one told me what to do. So, then I said, "Do you find that understanding humoral theory a bit better helps you to choose herbs for your patient?" He said, "No." I said, "Oh, so what's the point of it, why apply it?" and he said, "The point of humoral medicine is to make the doctor think that they understand the patient so they don't panic." And I said, "Well OK, how do you choose your herbs?" He said, "By intuition, doesn't everybody?" Informed intuition, of course, I mean, we don't just do it blind.

When with patients

When with patients, look closely and listen closely. They will tell you what's wrong with them. Listen longer and they'll tell you what to do about it. And then they pay you! It helps if you have white hair and look deep into their eyes. They will think you are wise![6]

The third floor of the Natural History Museum

Over here we tell students that the whole third floor of the Natural History Museum is occupied by people whose only aim is to make life difficult for herbalists. Seems to me that science is right only when it agrees with my grandmother. At first glance, all this re-ordering of

---

[6] Of course, Christopher was definitely wise, which is what makes this particularly humorous. [Ed.]

plants into different families is more consistent with traditional views of the plants than more modern views of herbal medicine, which, as a traditionalist, I find very encouraging. *Rhinanthus minor*, Yellow Rattle, has the same indications as Eyebright in traditional English herbal medicine. So, I can agree with the botanists here. Plantain and Foxglove sounds a bit outrageous though, but then I only know the genus Plantago. Is there a giant tropical Plantain with Foxglove-like flowers used for Elephant Fly bites perhaps? I do need some sort of consistent story here for my students. Pity about splitting up *Digitalis* species and Figworts, but then I suppose they couldn't take Scrophularia out of the Scrophulariaceae. Cardiac glycosides don't seem to be choosy but I would miss that bit of the story. I'll go with putting Veronica species with Plantain, since they have much feeling in common.

A very good understanding of biochemistry

A modern "scientific" medical approach works very well if we consider the whole of it. The failure of mainstream medicine is to focus on defined pathologies and ignore the underlying science. I teach my students to forget pathology and focus on physiology. We can clearly see how herbs interact with physiology—Physiomedical practice being, at its best, a good example. Use the herbs to address wrongness at a physiological level (or, even better, at a biochemical level) and there you are! Plants have a very good understanding of biochemistry and can easily deduce how to help to correct an imbalance in the physiological processes they are presented with.

Make a tea

If a plant jumps out at you, you must make a tea.

Pushed down

In the European tradition (and no doubt in everyone else's), joy nourishes the liver and any negative emotion damages it. The liver stores emotions. I had a patient once who told me that some years previously she had been rushed into hospital with acute jaundice. All tests proved negative and she slowly got better during her stay. She never understood why but patients will tell you everything in time. It turned out that she was in a relationship with a violent man and had to keep all her anger and strong emotions under control—pushed down into her liver. She also told me that she had asthma as a child and it was cured by taking her into the fields when the Gorse was being burnt off. In a moment of inspiration, I made some Gorse smudge sticks—I only ever tried this once and didn't use any on patients in case they asked for more.

Anybody could have done it

I had a client a few years ago who had an accident, I always tell this story to beginning herbalists because it shows just how nice simple things work. He'd broken his leg and scarred the artery, so the artery had healed up with a kink in it, so there wasn't any blood coming to his foot, you could see it, it was quite amazing. He took his sock off and he was pink down so far and then white below, and he liked to walk a lot and he couldn't walk because he was getting pain in the foot after about one hundred yards or so because of the oxygen not getting down to the muscles there. And the sad thing about it was that he'd spent two years since the accident going back and forth and back and forth to the hospital, the hospital couldn't actually do anything. And when the hospitals can't actually do anything, they have a test don't they? They say, "I know, let's give him a test." And he had all these tests including the doppler ultrasound. I like that, it always reminds me of school physics lessons about trains—the doppler effect and the trains coming towards you and then sounding different as they're going away from you. Something to do with that. And they said to him, they said, "Well, your circulation", having spent all this money, "your circulation isn't getting below the old scar." Now he was a professional man. He was a psychotherapist, he wasn't easily brow beaten or anything, but he was totally brow beaten by the whole experience and he was depressed and his friend made him come and see me and basically all we did was we gave him Hawthorn internally, to help heal the arteries, and a hot oil[7] to rub in and in three months he was walking. But the nice thing about

---

[7] This could easily have been "Non's hot oil"—a macerated oil made with Cayenne pepper, Mustard powder, Ginger and Black Pepper. See Christopher Hedley and Non Shaw, *Herbal Remedies* (Parragon, 1996), 61. For other possibilities, see Christopher Hedley and Non Shaw, *The Herbal Book of Making & Taking* (London: Aeon Books, 2020). [Ed.]

that is of course anybody could have done it, you don't need to be a professional herbalist to have done that, his sister could have done it, his granny could have done it, anybody could have done it, the lady in the shop down the end of the road could have done it, just look at his foot and say, "Ah right, it's cold, let's rub some hot stuff in."

The plants themselves

I find that I gain a lot from practitioners from any part of the world provided that we base our discussion on the plants themselves and use very simple or poetic language for pathology. The point is to get "below" such concepts as yin, kapha, melancholy, etc., even to get below such basic concepts as fire and water. If I base my discussion in any particular "system", I automatically limit how much I can learn. If we simply hang out with the plants, not only am I taking part in my own healing (which is the only valid reason for taking up medicine in the first place), I am setting no limits to how much I can learn—other than those imposed by the human condition itself.

It won't let me use it

Enchanter's Nightshade grows in my garden as you say as a weed, and it won't let me actually use it. And I think, at the moment anyway maybe I just need to grow it a bit more, get to know it a bit more and a bit more. I keep planning and I keep thinking there is a person who I could give Enchanter's Nightshade. One of the Saxon indications for Enchanter's Nightshade was what they called "wéden-heort", which is madness with frenzy in the heart. But, no, it won't let me use it.

The way she uses the herb

It's a thing I always noticed, seeing it happen to me as well when I was a herbal student. I went round different herbalists and some herbalists would say that this is a great herb for this, another herbalist would say that it doesn't work. And that's just because that's just the way that those people have used those herbs, the way those people relate to those herbs. Whether or not they're friends with those herbs, bottom line. I remember my teacher when I was training, I call her my teacher because when I was training at the college I used to go into her dispensary. I had to do dispensing, look after the patients, reception work, looking up files, all that sort of thing. Gardening, cutting the climbing Rose back which is something which will forever stick in my memory as a vicious climbing Rose. My teacher was well known for treating multiple sclerosis and she used a whole range of nervines. Certainly, St John's wort, Passiflora, Skullcap, Oats a lot, that sort of thing. Obvious things, like you would for treating multiple sclerosis. And one day when I was in there, a famous herbalist sent her a letter and she said, "Oh look, he's sent me this letter and it says, 'I've been having great success in multiple sclerosis using Primrose flowers.'" Use Primrose flowers as a nervine? Nice, quite a nice little nervine. And so, she started using Primrose flowers and all her patients stopped getting better. And then she said, "Well, it doesn't work. It doesn't work for me. It works for him." This isn't anything to do with magic. It's to do with the way she uses the herb, the combinations of the herbs, the way she understands the herb, the type of person that she gives that particular herb to. Though she always called it magic. So, different herbs work for different people.

Even you and me

All herbs have a story
There are many aspects to that story
Many people add to it
Everyone who uses, grows, prepares or picks the herb adds to it
Even phytotherapists[8]
Even traditional people
Our ancestors sang the songs which make up the hearts of these stories
Traditional people still do

The story of every herb changes, grows, contracts, expands, deepens
As people interact with that herb
Even you and me

The interaction becomes the story
The story becomes the interaction

---

[8] A herbalist was originally named here, who would likely identify themselves as a "phytotherapist". [Ed.]

As far as healing with herbs goes, the story *is* the healing

There exists a class of people whose lives constantly add to these stories Let's call these people herbalists

Slingbacks or open-toed sandals

Every practitioner needs a philosophy. Not the rules which define conditions and determine the most suitable herbal remedy (this is objective and cross cultural to some extent), but to explain why they feel the need to be a herbalist at all. This cannot, and should not, be unified. It would be like making only one size of shoes. We can all agree on the benefit of a philosophy, just as we can all agree on the benefits of wearing shoes, but one size would pinch some and be too big for others. Badly fitting philosophies, like shoes, lead to bunions and callouses. We need several sizes, even styles—some people might like a little height or be more comfortable in slingbacks or open-toed sandals. Enough variety so that we can all walk comfortably. So, we need to have a personal philosophy, a criterion of being (not a justification for action), with an ethos, an inbuilt awareness, and be accepting of responsibility. It should be flexible and wide, able to expand with experiences, and it should be strengthening and life enhancing.

Make it up as you go along

The only reason you do a herbal medicine course is to give yourself the confidence to be able to make it up as you go along. And this must be the case, mustn't it? It must be the case because if you're treating a patient, you're treating that person in front of you and that person in front of you is there for then and that's it and you're trying to treat the whole person, and if they come back next time they're going to be a different person, so you're going to have to make up something, aren't you? So, it's absolutely true you just make it up as you go along.

Two rules in herbal medicine

Having said that, there are actually two rules in herbal medicine. The first rule is label everything. I still have bottles in the back of my kitchen that one day I am going to remember what is in them. I'm going to remember that one day. I'll wake up one morning and go, "Oh! Starwort!" or something. The other rule is never eat anything until you see me eat it first and have waited a bit. Never eat anything until you've seen me eat it first, or your teacher, and waited a bit, just to be on the safe side. Mind you, herbalists are notorious for eating all sorts of things just to see what will happen, aren't they? So, there you go. Oh, and there's a subsection to that rule isn't there? Which a lot of herbalists use, which is Rule 2 subsection "a"—especially umbellifers, yes? You know your botany, you know that family is a very tricky family. And it's difficult to tell them apart. Do you have Hemlock Water Dropworts here? I'm sure you have similar species, it grows in the river, it grows in the canal by me. Some people say that it is the most poisonous plant in England, don't know how you'd prove it. It tastes and looks exactly like Celery when it's just coming up, I've even picked it myself and thought, "Oh! Celery". I remember walking down the canal thinking, "Oh! Celery" and then thinking, "Ah, mmm, good job I haven't swallowed that yet." Hemlock Water Dropwort.

Become a different person

If it is done really well and if the patient is open enough then it is only necessary to support the patient. A good example being the first cancer patient I ever knew, long before I accepted that I was a herbalist, who was "cured" by God—she was converted to a Pentecostal church. I draw inspiration from this and tell my patients that the only true way to beat cancer (or, indeed any serious disease, or indeed any disease) is to become a different person. If you become a different person then you can't have the same diseases. Becoming different means changing every aspect of your life—spiritual, emotional and physical.

All that matters

Tastes and temperatures of herbs are best appreciated by tasting and feeling. I always tell students that this is basically a creative writing exercise and that they should say exactly what they actually taste or feel. In this way I will always get a disagreement and then I can say that everyone's experience of a herb is different and all that matters is that we work on extending our own, unique appreciation of each herb.

Shut both eyes

It's really nice to do blind tasting in a group. And if you do double blind tasting, you shut both eyes. So, you get a group to taste the herb and to write down their impressions of it—the "energetics", if you like, the feeling of the herb within their body. You learn a lot that way, it's quite amazing what you learn, most especially from absolute beginners. There's actually three levels to this exercise, you taste the herb and you see how it tastes and you write down the impressions. And it's basically a creative writing exercise, it's best to use ordinary terms and trying to avoid scientific terms. The taste of the herb is just part of it, the next part is the appropriation, the part of the body which the herb likes to go to. If you meditate with a herb, you feel it going somewhere and doing things inside. And the last part of the exercise is to say, "It is like", because that's bringing the sensations into reality, you say, "It is like", and you say it is like I don't know, a film star or a friend of yours or a colour or whatever, people will come up with different things. You can just taste the tea and then you start the sentence. It's really interesting to do it in a group, especially with a group of people who've got to know each other, because different constitutions respond in different ways. And the fiery people will say such and such about the herb, and the earthy people will say such and such about the herb. This means the group get to know a little bit about the different ways you can use the herb with different people.

Your own

I always think that if you go and sit in with a herbalist with thirty years' experience, as a student, and you can understand anything they're talking about, then they're probably no good. Because by the end of thirty years, you've made the whole thing your own.

Best medicine

I think, weeds in a way must make the best medicine because they're the herbs that come around with us, aren't they? They follow us around saying, "OK, you need me! You need me!" Do you like that trick that the old herbalists used to say, that "If you look in someone's garden, you can see what they need"?

You just describe it

We learn from asking the herb, from contemplating how it is in the world and from tasting it, and then from watching its interactions with patients. That's what patients are for, of course, to help you learn about herbs, that's right isn't it? This should be the main source of our knowledge, our trunk. We can also extend our understanding by looking to its roots, to the history of the whole plant, to the plant's interaction with humanity as a whole, to its story. After I finished the herb course, I thought I'd give myself a treat, you need a treat after you've finished that, don't you? It's bloody hard work. And I went and did a story telling course, it was actually one of the most useful things, I went to the story telling course and, of course, people go to evening classes just to meet other people and have cups of coffee, don't they? That's what they do, so they're always chattering away to each other. And the storyteller came in and she sat down and didn't say anything at all, and the whole place went quiet. And she said the way you tell a story is you store it up into your mind so you can visualise it, and you just describe it. And that's what she did, that's what she taught me. It's great with patients, of course, because a patient is someone who's sick, whose life story has been interrupted by illness, and what you're doing is you're trying to re-thread the story, to join it up again. So, storytelling, it's a useful thing, I think. So, we learn from the history, and we can learn from the roots, and we can also learn from the branches. The very tip of the branch as I see it is maybe modern research, it's coming out and coming up into time. And modern research is the least useful source of information on herbs, although it does sometimes throw a light on your traditional knowledge. Basically, if you read research on a herb and it contradicts traditional knowledge, then the research is wrong. Although, you can usually find out where it went wrong and you can usually see that.

I want to be a Victorian vicar

In my next incarnation, I want to be a Victorian vicar. You know, someone with one of those small parishes, basically just the private parish of Lady so and so, so there's just the family's births and weddings and funerals, maybe two parishioners, and you have lots of time to go out and look around the countryside and count butterflies and whatever. That's what I'm going to do.

Egg-sucking

In my opinion, there is no substitute for making your own medicines yourself; although, I do allow buying from small businesses where you have direct contact with the people who actually handle the herbs. Close knowledge of the herb itself is an imperative, but we should not neglect close knowledge of the medicine maker as well. At the risk of lecturing my granny on egg-sucking, herbal medicine is built up from the intent of the herb itself (as a being in the world), the intent of the person who makes a medicine from that plant (as a gardener, farmer, cook, pharmacist, whatever), the intent of the herbalist supplying it, and the interaction between that accumulated intent and the patient's internal processes. We neglect any of these stages at our peril.

Studying the herb itself

The other thing we all learn at herb school was herbs have actions, but that's rubbish isn't it? Herbs don't have actions, have you seen a Dandelion rushing around the garden crying, "Diuresis! diuresis!" I haven't. Herbs have interactions, they interact with a person, which is, of course, why different people will respond to different herbs and that's the real trick isn't it, finding the herb to fit the person and that's really the use of energetics to find the herb to fit the person. And it gets really jolly good results. If you want to use a term similar to actions, I actually like the old-fashioned term "virtues". It implies something specific and essential about the being of the herb itself. So, when we study energetics, it isn't the actions of the herbs or its constituents, I think we're studying the herb itself.

In search of a trunk

My main teachers called themselves Physiomedicalists and they used the polypharmacy system which had been developed in the British Physiomedical tradition. This often involved thirty or forty herbs in a prescription, took an age to dispense and relied on a profound understanding of synergy. Being drawn to herbal medicine by the plants themselves, I looked to using more simple formulae, from which I hoped to learn about the virtues of the plants as individuals, rather than as members of a team. No one told me that I could learn directly from the plants themselves—although the concept lurked in my mind as it seemed intrinsic to Culpeper's method and he was my original inspiration. Culpeper liked simples and the constituent chemistry people went for simple formulae. Thus, I evolved a system with traditional roots and phytochemical branches—and have spent the next twenty odd years trying to find a trunk.

Up until that point

I went down to a herb conference years and years and years ago and we were staying in this cottage with a group of other herbalists. I got up in the morning early because the bloody birds were singing, and I went out for a walk and I found, believe it or not, Herb Christopher. I found Herb Christopher. Now Herb Christopher (*Actaea spicata*), as you probably know, only grows in Yorkshire and we were in Devon. But I convinced myself it was Herb Christopher and so I thought that it will be really good for me so I rushed home, got some water, put it in water. I'd found Herb Christopher! And when everybody got up, I said, "You must come and see what I've found, you must come and see what I've found!" We had bendle with us and he said, "How can I put this? That's not Herb Christopher." And then all of a sudden it turned into Sanicle (*Sanicula europaea*). It was Herb Christopher up until that point. So, I use Sanicle primary for people who have deluded themselves.

Storing sunsets

Years and years ago a herbalist brought over this Guatemalan herbalist, that was in the days before the Americans destroyed Guatemala. And we showed him around some herbally places, and then we took him to some touristy places, took him to Covent Garden, and he says, "Oh Covent Garden is touristy, but it's not actually much fun is it really?" And he said, "Where's the place where you can see the best sunset?", and we thought we'll go to Waterloo Bridge, that's the place to see the best sunset in London, Waterloo Bridge. So, we took him to Waterloo Bridge to watch the sun go down, and he said, "What's the English word for that place in your heart where you store things?" Hmmm. He went round the world because he was a representative for the Guatemalan government, he went round the world storing sunsets in his heart. He said, "I'll tell you where the best place to see sunsets."

It's in Korea apparently, you might like to know that, over the big river in Korea. Storing sunsets, that's a thing to do.[9]

How the plant is in the world

What we're interested in is how the plant is, how the plant is in the world, because how the plant is in the world, is how it will be in your body, when you take it. I always like to give Nettle as a good example, we can all think about Nettles, can't we? I don't have to bring one with me, do I? I was told a long time ago by a herbalist that I shouldn't actually talk about plants behind their back. Thought, that's nice. You have to forgive us, Nettle. So, how is Nettle in the world? Where does it grow? It grows around human beings because it likes rich soil and human beings make sure the soil is rich, so it'll grow down the bottom of the cow field where the cows have been and on your compost heap of course. It likes really rich soil, it grows around humans. And growing round humans is a fairly dangerous occupation. But I think Nettles have a wonderful solution to this, they sting you and the sting contains various substances including histamine, which is the main warning chemical used by mammals. How does Nettle know that? Must have been reading books. So, basically it makes you jump and its bark is worse than its bite. It hurts but it doesn't kill you, so you don't rip it up, which I think is incredibly clever strategy don't you? And of course, if you take a Nettle inside that's what it does, it prickles things and gets things moving, gets things going.

How it be

Some people have used the word "energetics" here, not totally sure what I think about that word. It seems to be simply a way of trying to express how the plants act in our bodies—hot and cold, wet and dry, moving and stabilising, dispersing, consolidating and so on. But actually, all this arises from how the plant is in the world, how it be, as Granny Weatherwax might say, do you know Terry Pratchett's Granny Weatherwax? "It doesn't matter what you do, what matters is how

---

[9] I recently found out that Liz Oldham—educator, herbalist, friend and colleague of Christopher's, who proofread this volume, as well as being the author of the wonderful newsletter "Flourish"—also stores sunsets. I hope it's catching. [Ed.]

you be." And it's by looking at the plant and seeing how it is, how it be in the world, that you get that, that's how it starts to tell you things.

Adopting ancestors

Picking the berries with my friend, up on Hampstead Heath, this year I was aware, as so often before, of the old people picking with us. My friend is African, he says the ancestors are all around us all the time. We joked that they probably hang around waiting for a living person to start on a traditional occupation so they can join in. Do they lurk in gangs at the bottom of Willow Road, watching the Elder trees and getting excited when someone walks up the road carrying a large, empty bag? I think they do. Of late, I have come to the conclusion that we can adopt ancestors in this way, no matter what our lineage. Herbal medicine can be carried out in a traditional manner. If we do so then there are plenty of ancestors with good heart waiting to support us, no matter what our lineage.

Ineffable mystery

I am a Virgo and well understand the joys of classification—and its limitations. I too have played with East/West comparisons. I too have drawn up charts and studied traditional systems. I have come to the conclusion that every patient is an ineffable mystery and any system of classification I use is basically for my own benefit, to give me an angle and a possible direction. When I become wedded to any particular interpretation of the mystery in front of me, then I let my patient down.

More baggy here

Well, the Chinese like to store things in boxes, don't they. The Japanese like that too, beautiful little packages. Their information is all tidied up in categories. So, it's easier to see it and catalogue it. Like a library. And Ayurveda is similar, things have boundaries, their knowledge is organised. We're just far more baggy here, constitutionally. We're more like the plants themselves in the way we think and remember. Our stories are more sprawling and vine-like, so our way of passing on knowledge is more like the plants too. Seeds and runners.

I shouldn't worry

I shouldn't worry. There will always be herbalists. As long as there are plants and there are people, there will be herbalists. All the information you need, all the knowing is in the plants themselves. It's a question of accessing that information, isn't it? And herbalists are the ones who know how to talk to the plants and how to ask them to share their information with the people. And if you know how to talk to the plants, you'll always have access to the information, won't you. All the systems and models and theories are only ways to catalogue and systemise that information so that humans can refer back to it.

Most together

I am reminded that a few years ago I treated a young man diagnosed as schizophrenic. At the time, I was working with Hildegard von Bingen's recipes which always include lots of spices. We tried a number of variations. I was taken by Calamus because I have read that it is used in India to clear the mind—and indeed it does. This was the herb that he found most helpful. Mind you, during treatment he moved to a Hare Krishna community and was given charge of their sacred oxen. He said that this was the time when he was most together—you can't act mad with an ox, they simply ignore you.

One degree under

My understanding is that current thought is coming around to the traditional view. That rhinoviruses thrive when the blood supply to the respiratory mucosa is diminished. It is a frequent observation in practice that cold individuals often develop respiratory tract infections when chilled and that a good strong cup of Ginger and Cinnamon or inhalation of steam will prevent this. I myself am an example. This was my grandmother's opinion and my grandmother's medical judgements have never been proved wrong. In cold weather blood should come to the surface initially and only retreat when the cold increases but if the constitution is cold then blood retreats too quickly, the nose gets cold and the viruses thrive. People with upper respiratory tract viral infection often prove to be one degree under—this is a useful diagnostic tool. So, it seems to me that these viruses, once they have a hold will tend to lower the body temperature in order to consolidate their hold on the system. Clever! It is also noticeable that, in cold constitutions, cold weather will cause the nose to run. To me this is a protective measure, also quite smart.

Get below

Not being especially sharp, I like to make simple pictures for myself, and for my students. My picture of the immune system (apart from noting that it is more like an anarchists' collective than an army) is a "black box" full of all sorts of cells and chemicals. Disease penetrates into the immune system. The depth of penetration depends on the aggressiveness of the condition and the weakness of the patient's constitution. The main plank of herbal treatment is to get below the disease. I can't get my head around the difference between, say, immunomodulators and immune tonics, so I prefer to simply focus on how deep in the immune system a herb works. I suppose that relates to how nourishing an immune herb is. My teaching technique is to get the students to say how deep is the place from which any given herb moves to support the immune system and I haven't made any definitive tables but it would be quite nice to give them one. As a starting point, here is my roughly thought-out table—as with all tables it runs the risk of doing the listed herbs no real justice but, still, I have to start somewhere. The list is from most superficial, at the top, to most deep, at the bottom.

Elderflowers
Yarrow
Cayenne
Ephedra
Echinacea
Astragalus
Elderberries
Boneset
Ground ivy
Thuja
Garlic
Garden Sage
St John's wort
Panax ginseng

Baikal Skullcap
Artemisia spp.
Siberian ginseng
Ashwagandha
Rehmannia
Borage
Elecampane
Burdock
Liquorice
Ganoderma spp.
Turkey tail
Antioxidant foods—EFAs, berries, carrot juice, beetroot juice, brassicas, green tea etc. (including supplements and spices taken in reasonable amounts)

The idea is that diseases penetrate the body more or less deeply. The depth of penetration depends on a number of factors including the aggressiveness of the disease vector and the cohesion and integrity of the immune system. The relevance to prescription formulation is that a prescription must reach a point underneath[10] the disease in order to expel it. For example, Elderflowers and Eyebright will work well for many cases of hay fever but if the person's immune system is severely run down then herbs which go deeper, such as Baikal Skullcap or even *Ganoderma* spp., will be needed.

Really

Very generous things, plants—we don't deserve them, really.

---

[10] Although Christopher doesn't mention it here, I suspect that he might also have added that a prescription should get "just" underneath the disease, rather like scooping a fish out of water: if you are too far below the fish, it will sense you and get away, but if you are "just" below, you have a better chance of having fish for dinner. Similarly, you might have to get underneath but as close to the disease as possible for you to have the best chance of landing the disease on the riverbank, where it can do no harm. [Ed.]

REFERENCES

Barker, Julian. *The Medicinal Flora of Britain & Northwest Europe.* West Wickham, Kent: Winter Press, 2001.

Baumann, Andre, Marisa Skaljac, Rüdiger Lehmann, Andreas Vilcinskas, and Zdeněk Franta. "Urate Oxidase Produced by Lucilia sericata Medical Maggots Is Localized in Malpighian Tubes and Facilitates Allantoin Production." *Insect Biochemistry and Molecular Biology* 83 (April 1, 2017): 44–53. https://doi.org/10.1016/j.ibmb.2017.02.007.

Beeton, Isabella. *Mrs. Beeton's Book of Household Management: The 1861 Classic with Advice on Cooking, Cleaning, Childrearing, Entertaining, and More.* Western Classics, 2020.

Bennett, Bradley C. "Doctrine of Signatures: Through Two Millennia." *HerbalGram*, no. 78 (2008): 34–45. https://www.herbalgram.org/resources/herbalgram/issues/78/table-of-contents/article3244/.

Bone, Kerry, and Simon Mills. *Principles and Practice of Phytotherapy: Modern Herbal Medicine.* 2nd ed. Edinburgh Churchill Livingstone, Elsevier, 2013.

British Herbal Medicine Association. Scientific Committee. *British Herbal Pharmacopoeia, 1983.* London: British Herbal Medicine Association, 1983.

Burton, Robert. *The Anatomy of Melancholy.* 1652. Reprint, London: Chatto and Windus, 1883. https://www.exclassics.com/anatomy/anatomy1.pdf.

Cheetham, Tom. *Imaginal Love*. Spring Publications, 2015.

Cockayne, Thomas Oswald, Barbarus Apuleius, Sextus Placitus, and Dioscorides. *Leechdoms, Wortcunning, and Starcraft of Early England. Being a Collection of Documents, for the Most Part Never before Printed, Illustrating the History of Science in This Country before the Norman Conquest*. Longman, Green, Longman, Roberts, and Green, 1864. https://archive.org/details/leechdomswortcun02cock/page/n7/mode/2up.

Cook, William. H. *The Physiomedical Dispensatory*. Wm. H. Cook, 1869. https://www.henriettes-herb.com/eclectic/cook/index.html.

Culpeper, Nicholas. *Culpeper's Complete Herbal*. 1653. Reprint, Wordsworth Reference, 1995.

Culpeper, Nicholas. *The English Physician Enlarged: With Three Hundred and Sixty Nine Medicines, Made of English Herbs, That Were Not in Any Impression until This*. London: W. Baynes, 1799. https://wellcomecollection.org/works/tazb4r8a/items.

Ellingwood, Finley. *American Materia Medica, Therapeutics and Pharmacognosy*. Ellingwood's Therapeutist, 1919. https://wellcomecollection.org/works/jt4unq8f/items.

Felter, Harvey Wickes, and John Uri Lloyd. *King's American Dispensatory*. Cincinnati: Ohio Valley Co., 1898. https://www.henriettes-herb.com/eclectic/kings/intro.html.

Gerard, John. *The Herball or Generall Historie of Plantes*. London: John Norton, 1597. http://www.biolib.de/gerarde/gerarde_herball.pdf.

The Grete Herball Whiche Geueth Parfyt Knowlege and Vnderstandyng of All Maner of Herbes [And] There Gracyous Vertues Whiche God Hath Ordeyned for Our Prosperous Welfare and Helth, for They Hele [And] Cure All Maner of Dyseases and Sekenesses That Fall or Mysfortune to All Maner of Creatoures of God Created, Practysed by Many Expert and Wyse Maysters, as Auicenna [And] Other. [Et]C. Also It Geueth Full Parfyte Vnderstandynge of the Booke Lately Prentyd by Me (Peter Treueris) Named the Noble Experiens of the Vertuous Handwarke of Surgery. London: Peter Treveris, 1526. https://quod.lib.umich.edu/e/eebo2/A03048.0001.001/1:21?rgn=div1;view=toc.

Grieve, Maud. *A Modern Herbal*. Vol. 2. 1931. Reprint, Dover Publications, 1971.

Grimes, Ronald. "Performance Is Currency in the Deep World's Gift Economy: An Incantatory Riff for a Global Medicine Show." In *The Handbook of Contemporary Animism*, edited by Graham Harvey, 501–12. London: Routledge, 2013.

Ha, Sha. "A Review on Medicine in Medieval Times and the Multicultural Origin and Development of the Salerno Medical School." *Medicina Historica* 6, no. 2 (2022): e2022021. https://www.mattioli1885journals.com/index.php/MedHistor/article/view/11319/10937.

Hatfield, Gabrielle. *Memory, Wisdom, and Healing: The History of Domestic Plant Medicine*. Alan Sutton Publishing, 1999.

Hedley, Christopher, and Non Shaw. *Herbal Remedies*. Paragon, 1996.

———. *A Herbal Book of Making and Taking*. London: Aeon Books, 2020.

———. *Plant Medicine—a Collection of the Teachings of Herbalists Christopher Hedley and Non Shaw*. Edited by Guy Waddell. London: Aeon Books, 2023.

Hobbs, Christopher. *Christopher Hobbs's Medicinal Mushrooms: The Essential Guide*. Storey Publishing, LLC, 2021.

———. *Medicinal Mushrooms*. Botanica Press, 1996.

Holmes, Peter. *The Energetics of Western Herbs: A Materia Medica Integrating Western and Chinese Herbal Therapeutics*. Vol. 1. Boulder, Colo.: Snow Lotus Press, 2007.

Kooser, Ted, and Jim Harrison. *Braided Creek*. Copper Canyon Press, 2023.

Lad, Vasant. *Ayurveda—the Science of Self-Healing: A Practical Guide*. Lotus Press, 1993.

Marder, Michael. *Green Mass—the Ecological Theology of St Hildegard of Bingen*. Stanford: Stanford University Press, 2021.

Mills, Simon. *The Essential Book of Herbal Medicine*. Penguin, 1993.

Mills, Simon, and Kerry Bone. *Principles and Practice of Phytotherapy: Modern Herbal Medicine*. Edinburgh: Churchill Livingstone, 2000.

Moller, Violet. *Map of Knowledge : How Classical Ideas Were Lost and Found—a History of Seven Cities*. London: Picador, 2020.

Paulus, Aegineta. *The Seven Books of Paulus Ægineta*. Translated by Francis Adams. Sydenham: Sydenham Society, 1884. https://www.gutenberg.org/ebooks/author/55793.

Priest, A.W. *Studies in Physiomedicalism. Paper 1. Historical and Philosophical*. A.W. Priest, 1959.

———. *Studies in Physiomedicalism. Paper 2. Principles of Diagnosis*. A.W. Priest, 1959.

———. *Studies in Physiomedicalism. Paper 3. Principles of Medication*. A.W. Priest, 1961.

———. *Studies in Physiomedicalism. Paper 4. Materia Medica*. A.W. Priest, 1962.

———. *Studies in Physiomedicalism. Paper 5. Principles of Therapeutics*. A.W. Priest, 1963.

Priest, A.W., and L. R. Priest. *Herbal Medication: A Clinical and Dispensary Handbook.* The C.W. Daniel Company Ltd, 2000.

Rumi. *Selected Poems.* Translated by Coleman Barks, John Moyne, A.J. Arberry, and Reynold Nicholson. London: Penguin, 2004.

Salmon, William. *Pharmacopoeia Londinensis, Or, the New London Dispensatory.* T. Baffett, R. Chifwell, M. Wotton, G. Conyers and I. Dawks, 1696. https://archive.org/details/bim_early-english-books-1641-1700_pharmacopoeia-londinensi_salmon-william_1696/page/28/mode/2up.

Sayyah, Mehdi, Hatam Boostani, Siroos Pakseresht, and Alireza Malayeri. "Comparison of Silybum Marianum (L.) Gaertn. With Fluoxetine in the Treatment of Obsessive–Compulsive Disorder." *Progress in Neuro-Psychopharmacology and Biological Psychiatry* 34, no. 2 (March 17, 2010): 362–65. https://doi.org/10.1016/j.pnpbp.2009.12.016.

Scholl, Philip, Douglas Colwell, and Ramón Cepeda-Palacios. "Myiasis (Muscoidea, Oestrodea)." In *Medical and Veterinary Entomology*, edited by Gary Mullen and Lance Durden, 384–419. Elsevier Inc., 2019.

Schwarzstein, Marco André, ed. *Imaginal Worlds.* Thompson, Connecticut: Spring Publications, 2023.

Strehlow, Wighard. *Hildegard of Bingen's Spiritual Remedies.* Rochester, Vt.: Healing Arts Press, 2002.

Taylor, Stephen. *The Humoral Herbal.* London: Aeon Books, 2021.

Waddell, Guy. "The Matter of Knowing Plant Medicine as Ecology—from Vegetal Philosophy and Plant Science to Tea Tasting in the Anthropocene." In *Plants Matter*, edited by Luci Attala and Louise Steel, 135–59. Cardiff: University of Wales Press, 2023.

Wasson, Robert Gordon. *Soma: Divine Mushroom of Immortality.* Harcourt Brace Jovanovich, 1968. https://www.en.psilosophy.info/pdf/soma_divine_mushroom_of_immortality_(psilosophy.info).pdf.

Weiss, Rudolf Fritz. *Herbal Medicine.* Arcanum, 1988.

West, Cornel. *Hope on a Tightrope.* Smiley Books, 2008.

Yoors, Jan. *The Gypsies.* Waveland Press, 1987.

INDEX

Note: page numbers in **bold** indicate major herb entries with their own headings. Page numbers followed by (f) indicate that the content will be found in a footnote on that page.

Achillea millefolium, see Yarrow
Achillea ptarmica, see Sneezewort
Acorus calamus, see Calamus
Actaea spicata, see Herb Christopher
Adenosine triphosphate, xxi
adopting ancestors, 111
Agrimony (*Agrimonia eupatoria*), 55
air, *see* sanguine humour
Alchemilla vulgaris, A. mollis, see Lady's Mantle
alchemists, 61, 97
allantoin, 33–34, 34 (f)
Allium sativum, see Garlic
Amanita muscaria, see Fly Agaric
Angelica (*Angelica archangelica*), 18
Anthemis cotula, see Mayweed
anticholinergic effect, 30
antioxidant foods, 114
applying basic principles, 101–102

Arctium lappa, see Burdock root
Artemisia absinthium, see Wormwood
Artemisia vulgaris, see Mugwort
Artichokes (*Cynara scolymus*), 21, 66
Artist's Bracket (*Ganoderma applanatum*), **27–28**
Astragalus (*Astragalus mongholicus* syn. *A. membranaceus*), xxv, **29**
Ayurveda—the Science of Self-Healing: A Practical Guide (Lad), 14

Ballota nigra, see Black Horehound
Balm, *see* Lemon Balm
Barberry (*Berberis vulgaris*), **49**
Barker, Julian, 30, 56
Beech (*Fagus sylvatica*), 28
Beeton, Isabella, 16
Berberis aquifolium, see Mahonia
Berberis vulgaris, see Barberry

120   INDEX

Betonica officinalis, see Wood Betony
bitters, 7
Bittersweet (*Solanum dulcamara*), **30**
Black Horehound (*Ballota nigra*), 97
Boneset (*Eupatorium perfoliatum*), **30–31**, 31 (f), 34 (f), 38 (f)
Borage (*Borago officinalis*), 6, 6 (f), **31**, 34 (f), 38 (f)
British Herbal Pharmacopeia, 49, 50
Brounstein, Howie, xx, xxx
Burdock root, 72

Calamus (*Acorus calamus*), 112
Calendula officinalis, see Marigold
Canadian Fleabane (*Conyza canadensis*), asking a question of, 98
Cayenne (*Capsicum annuum* syn. *C. frutescens*), **32**, 101 (f)
Chamomile (*Matricaria chamomilla*), 12
Chaste Berry (*Vitex agnus-castus*), **32–33**, 32 (f), 60
   dosage, 32–33
   impact on libido, 32
   improving lives, 33
   leaves, 33
cheese, 14
Chelidonium majus, see Greater Celandine
choleric humour, 3–8
   adolescence and shift from childhood vitality, 5
   becoming fiery, 23
   Boneset (*Eupatorium perfoliatum*), 30–31, 31 (f)
   burnt choler, 5–6
   clear thinkers, 8
   consolidating power of bitters, 7
   cooling needed, 8
   dominance of one humour in sickness, 8
   exercise, 5
   fire as doing, 22
   healing through self-awareness, 6
   relating to fiery temperaments, 6
   suppressed fire, 4, 6, 7
   traits and therapeutic approaches, 3–4

Cinnamon (*Cinnamomum* species), 17, 39, 41(f), 98, 112
Circaea lutetiana, see Enchanter's Nightshade
Cirsium acaule, see Dwarf thistle
Cirsium heterophyllum, see Melancholy Thistle
Clary Sage (*Salvia sclarea*) essential oil, 20
classification, limitations of, 111
Cockayne, Thomas Oswald, 39 (f), 40
Comfrey (*Symphytum officinale*), **33–34**, 38–39
   allantoin, 33–34
   cautions, 34 (f)
   deep tissue regeneration and traditional uses, 33–34
Commiphora molmol, see Myrrh
communicating with plants, 112
Coneflower, see Echinacea
connecting people with plants, 94
Convallaria majalis, see Lily of the Valley
Conyza canadensis, see Canadian Fleabane
Cook, William, 38
cordial, 29
Cramp Bark (*Viburnum opulus*), **35**
Crataegus species, see Hawthorn
crown shyness, xxvii
Culpeper, Nicholas, xxvi, xxix, 3, 6, 6 (f), 16, 18, 34, 39, 49, 61, 61 (f), 65, 71, 82, 82 (f), 91, 94, 94 (f), 99, 109
Curcuma longa, see Turmeric
Cynara scolymus, see Artichokes
cystic breasts, 85–86

Dandelion (*Taraxacum officinale*) 49, 74
depression, 88
   Hawthorn, 54–55
   Hops, 56
   Marigold, 97
   and melancholia, 19, 20
   Vitex, 33
diabetes, 45, 48
Dioscorides, xxiv
diuretic index of a herb, 72

doctrine of signatures, xxiv–xxvi, xxv (f)
dreaming, *see* Fly Agaric, Mugwort, St. John's Wort
dual humours, 22
Dwarf thistle (*Cirsium acaule*), 66

earth, *see* melancholy humour
Echinacea (*Echinacea* spp.), **35–37**
    in autoimmune conditions, 37
    combinations and alternatives, 35–36
    dosage, 35, 36
    E. pallida, 37
    E. purpurea, 36, 37
    septicaemia, 36
    steroids, 36
    and vitality, 36–37
Elderberries (*Sambucus nigra fructus*), 35
Elderflowers (*Sambucus nigra flos*), 36
Elecampane (*Inula helenium*), **37–40**
    in chicken stock, 40
    elfshot disease, 39–40
    in Greek mythology, 38
    lung diseases, 38–39
    as lung restorative, 38
    spleen herb, 38
elfshot disease, *see* Elecampane
ellagitannins, 55
Enchanter's Nightshade (*Circaea lutetiana*)
    and Elf disease, 40
    needing permission from, 102
energetics of herbs, xxx, 106, 108, 110–111
Ephedra (*Ephedra sinica*), **40–41**, 113
epilepsy, 73, 82
    paediatric, 65
Epilobium angustifolium, see Rosebay Willowherb
Equisetum arvense, see Horsetail
Essential Book of Herbal Medicine (Mills), 33
Eupatorium perfoliatum, see Boneset
Euphrasia officinalis, see Eyebright
European medicine, traditional, 96
Eyebright, xxv, 100, 114

Fairies, xx, xxiv, 59, 88, 93
Fennel (*Foeniculum vulgare*), 6 (f), 18, **41**, 41 (f)
Figwort (*Scrophularia nodosa* and *S. aquatica*), xxv, **41–42**, 100
Filipendula ulmaria, see Meadowsweet
fire, *see* choleric humour
Fireweed, *see* Rosebay Willowherb
first duty of a herbalist, 94
Fly Agaric (*Amanita muscaria*), **42–44**, 42 (f), 79
    dreaming visions, 43
    Fireweed and, 43–44
    as spiritual guide, 44
    toxicity, 42–43
Foeniculum vulgare, see Fennel
Fucus vesiculosus, see Kelp
fungal extracts, 28
fungi, medicinal, 27–28

Galen, xxix, 10
Galenic classification, xxix (f), xxxi, 13 (f), 57, 70, 83. *See also* choleric humour, melancholic humour, phlegmatic humour, sanguine humour
Ganoderma adspersum, see Shelf Fungus
Ganoderma applanatum, see Artist's Bracket
Ganoderma lucidum, see Reishi
Galega officinalis, see Goat's Rue
Garlic (*Allium sativum*), 21, 40, **44–46**
    arteriosclerosis, 45
    coughs and phlegm, 45–46
    diabetes, 45
    intermittent claudication, 44–45
"gay Socrates", xxi
Gentian (*Gentiana lutea*), 12
Geranium maculatum, see Spotted/Wild Geranium
Geum urbanum, see Herb Bennet
Ginkgo (*Ginkgo biloba*), **46–48**, 64
    blood clotting, 47–48
    dinosaurs, 46
    headaches, 47
    misgivings, 48

Ginseng (*Panax ginseng*), 113
Glechoma hederacea, see Ground Ivy
Goat's Rue (*Galega officinalis*), 48
Golden Seal (*Hydrastis canadensis*), xxv, 35, **49**
Greater Celandine (*Chelidonium majus*), xxv, 30, **50**
Greater Plantain (*Plantago major*), 74
Grete Herball, 82, 82 (f), 88
Grieve, Maud, 43, 50, 79 (f)
Grimes, Ronald, xxviii
Ground Ivy, 35
Guatemalan herbalist's wisdom, 109–110
gut astringents, 55–56

happy plants, 112
Harrison, Jim, xviii
Hawthorn (*Crataegus* spp.), 29, 48, **50–55**, 62, 76, 101
   addressing fear, 51–52
   Chinese berries versus Western berries, 52–53
   dosage, 52
   emotional healing, 54–55
   heart remedy, 53–54
   restorative power of, 54
   trophorestorative, 50–51
healing through becoming a different person, 105
heart failure, *see* Lily of the Valley
Hedley, Christopher, xvii–xxx
   calling to be a herbalist, xxiv, 93
   green grooviness and wisdom, xxi–xxiii
   humour, xxi
   narrative approaches of, xix–xx
   phytochemistry, tradition and plant intelligence, xxvi–xxvii
   reimagining of doctrine of signatures to include behaviour, xxiv–xxvi
   storytelling, xviii
   and vegetal philosophy, xxiii
Hemlock Water Dropwort (*Oenanthe crocata*), 105

Herb Bennet (*Geum urbanum*), **55–56**
   compared with other gut astringents, 55–56
   gut healing, 55
Herb Christopher (*Actaea spicata*), 109
Herbal Book of Making and Taking, A (Hedley and Shaw), xvii
Hildegard von Bingen, xxii, 41, 41 (f), 112
Hobbs, Christopher, 44, 44 (f)
Holmes, Peter, 58
Hops (*Humulus lupulus*), **56**
Horsetail (*Equisetum arvense*), **56–57**
   rebalancing of mineral metabolism, 56–57
   preparations, 57
humoral theory, function of, 99
humours, *see* choleric humour, melancholy humour, phlegmatic humour, sanguine humour
   comforting and calming, 23
   response by different humours to the same situation, 24
   transformation, 22–23
   two dominant humours, 22
Humulus lupulus, see Hops
Hydrastis canadensis, see Golden Seal
Hypericum perforatum, see St John's Wort

imaginal, xix
imaginal worlds, xx
immune system, 113
   fungal extracts in therapy, 27–28
   getting below the disease, 113–114
importance of listening, 97–98
importance of physiology over pathology, 100
intention, role of, 108
intuition in choosing herbs, xxiv, 99
Inula helenium, see Elecampane
Isatis tinctoria, see Woad

Juniper (*Juniperus communis*), xxiv, **57–58**

Kava kava (*Piper methysticum*), 72
Kelp (including *Fucus vesiculosus*), **58**
kidney stones, 72–73, 98
"King's evil". *See* scrophula
knowledge from speaking to plants, 98
Kooser, Ted, xviii

labelling and caution, 104–105
Lacquered Bracket (*Ganoderma resinaceum*), 27
Lady's Mantle (*Alchemilla vulgaris, A. mollis*), **58–61**
   alchemists, 61
   appearance, 58–59
   gynaecological uses, 59–60
   with other herbs, 60
   womb tonic as basis for use, 60
Laetiporus sulphureus, see Sulphur Polypore
Lamium purpureum, see Red Deadnettle
learning from how a plant is in the world, 110–111
learning through relating to plants, 102, 102–3, 103–4, 107
Leechbook of Bald, 39, 40
Lemon Balm (*Melissa officinalis*), 6, 6 (f), 18, **29–30**, 70
Leonurus cardiaca, see Motherwort
Lily of the Valley (*Convallaria majalis*), 52, **61–63**, 63 (f)
   disturbance of the Shen, 61
   dosage, 63
   heart failure, 61–63
Lime Flowers (*Tilia* spp.), flowering times of different species, **64**
liver decongestive, 21

Mahonia (*Berberis aquifolium*), **49**
making practice your own, 106
Mallows, 23, 38, 70, 70 (f)
Marigold (*Calendula officinalis*), 10, 60, 97
Matricaria chamomilla, see Chamomile
Mayweed (*Anthemis cotula*), **64**
mcdonald, jim, 20
Meadowsweet (*Filipendula ulmaria*), 47, 48

medicinal fungi, 28
Medicinal Mushrooms (Hobbs), 44
melancholy humour, 18–21
   being, 19, 20, 22
   being and creativity, 20–21
   earth, 22
   Eeyore, 18, 21
   melancholia versus depression, 19, 20
   melancholics and movement, 21
   Melilot, 18
   moving a stuck melancholic, 19–20
   moving, cleansing and warming herbs, 18, 19
   need for solitude, 19
   physical characteristics, 20, 21
   splenic, 19
   Thistles, 21, 65–66
   walking, 21
Melancholy Thistle (*Cirsium heterophyllum*), 21, 65
Melilot (*Melilotus officinalis*), 18
Melissa officinalis, see Lemon Balm
Mentha x piperita, see Peppermint
Milk Thistle (*Silybum marianum* syn. *Carduus marianus*), 43, 43 (f), **65–66**
   and other thistles for liver and treating melancholy, 65–66
   paediatric epilepsy, 65
   treating a racehorse, 65
Mills, Simon, 33
Mills, Simon, and Bone, Kerry, 47
miscarriages, 74, 83
Motherwort (*Leonurus cardiaca*), 6 (f), **66–67**, 77, 83
Mugwort (*Artemisia vulgaris*), **67–69**, 95
   catalyst and guide, 68
   dreaming practice, 67–68
   psychic protection, 68–69
   womb energiser, 67
multiple sclerosis, 103
mushroom extraction method, 28
Myrrh (*Commiphora molmol*), **69–70**

naming a plant as a magical act, 97
Nettle (*Urtica dioica*), **70–71**, 72, 110
new medicinal uses for plants, 95
Nietzsche, xxi
noticing an individual plant for the first time, 93

Oenanthe crocata, *see* Hemlock Water Dropwort
only two rules in herbal medicine, 104–105

Paeonia lactiflora, *see* Peony
Paget, Henry, 14 (f)
Panax ginseng, *see* Ginseng
Paracelsus, xxiv
Parietaria judaica, *see* Pellitory of the Wall
Passion Flower (*Passiflora incarnata*), 13, **72**
patients as mysteries, 111
Paulus, Aegineta, 96
Pearson, Nick, xxxi–xxxii
Pellitory of the Wall (*Parietaria judaica*), **72–73**
Peony (*Paeonia lactiflora*), **73**
people as donuts, 95
Pepper (*Piper nigrum*), 14
Peppermint (*Mentha x piperita*), **73**
Pharmacopoeia Londinensis (Salmon), 29
philosophy, need for, 104
phlegmatic humour, 13–18
    anger, 15
    balancing foods, 14
    Bittersweet, 30
    feelings and emotions, 22
    flowing and binding, 15
    Garlic (*Allium sativum*), 45–46
    lethargy, 17–18
    Nettle, 71
    overflowing phlegm, 13–14
    physical characteristics, 15, 16
    Piglet, 15
    rheumatism, 13–14
    the role of elders, 17
    temperament, 14
    water, 22–23
    working with phlegm, 16–17
physiomedicalism, 51, 51 (f), 90, 96, 96 (f), 100, 108
Phytolacca decandra, *see* Poke root
picking plants as ceremony, 93–94
pilgrimage, necessary suffering on, 94
Piper methysticum, *see* Kava kava
Piper nigrum, *see* Pepper
"plantabilities", xxvii
Plantain (*Plantago major, P. lanceolata*), **74–75**
    folk tales and fertility lore, 75
    verticality of, reflecting use, 74–75
Plant Medicine: A collection of the teachings of herbalists Christopher Hedley and Non Shaw (Hedley and Shaw), xvii, xviii, xxi, xxviii, xxix (f)
plant metabolites (primary and secondary), xxvi–xxvii
plant science, xxvi–xxvii
plant taxonomy changes, 99–100
Pliny the Elder, xxiv
Pointings, xx
Poke root (*Phytolacca decandra*), 36
Polypody of the Oak (*Polypodium vulgare*), **75**
the power of listening to patients, 99
practice as re-threading patient stories, 107
practice, the need to make it up, 104
Prickly Ash (*Zanthoxylum americanum, Z. clava-herculis*), **75–76**
Priest, A.W. and Priest, L. R., 51, 96
Priest, A.W., 58, 58 (f)
Principles and Practice of Phytotherapy: Modern Herbal Medicine (Mills and Bone), 1st Edition 2000; 2nd Edition (Bone and Mills) 2013, 47 (f)
Primrose flowers (*Primula vulgaris*), 103
prolactin-secreting tumours, 85
psychosomatic hypertension, 11–12
pyrrolizidine alkaloids, 31, 31 (f), 34, 34 (f), 38 (f)

Raspberry Leaf (*Rubus ideaus*), **76–78**
   colic, 77–78
   dried raspberries, 77–78
   womb tonic, 76–77
Red Clover (*Trifolium pratense*), 64
Red Deadnettle (*Lamium purpureum*), xxiii–xxiv, 93
Reishi (*Ganoderma lucidum*), 27
relaxant, in Physiomedicalism, 90
respiratory health, 112–113
Rheum officinale, R. palmatum, see Rhubarb
rheumatism, 13–14
rhinoviruses, 112
Rhubarb (*Rheum officinale, R. palmatum*), 78
Ribwort Plantain (*Plantago lanceolata*), **74**
Rose (*Rosa* spp.), **78–79**
Rosebay Willowherb (*Epilobium angustifolium*), 43–44, **79**
Rosemary (*Salvia rosmarinus* syn. *Rosmarinus officinalis*), **79–81**
   restorative for circulation, 79–80
   Hungarian Rosemary water, 80–81
   for remembrance, 81
Rubus ideaus, see Raspberry Leaf
Rumi, xxxii

Sage (*Salvia officinalis*), **81–86**
   acetylcholine-sparing effect, 82
   with Betony for Alzheimer's disease, 82
   cystic breasts, 85–86
   empty heat, 82
   grief and sorrow, 83
   holding the centre, 81–82
   Mayday tradition of Wild Sage gathering, 86
   memory, 85
   menopausal heat, 83
   mouth ulcers, 84
   prolactin-secreting tumours, 85
   smudging, 86
   total capacity point, 84–85
   traditional ways of using, 84
   warmth and dryness of, 83–84

Salmon, William, 29
Salvia officinalis, see Sage
Salvia rosmarinus syn. *Rosmarinus officinalis, see* Rosemary
Salvia sclarea, see Clary Sage
Sambucus nigra, see Elderberries, Elderflowers
sanguine humour, 8–13
   air, 22
   being authoritative as treatment strategy, 9
   better with age, 9
   in childhood, 8–9
   child-like and childish, 12
   herbs for, 13
   indulgence, 11, 12
   managing airy temperaments, 9–10
   managing somatic tension, 11–12
   tendency to be scattered, 10
   thinking, 22
   Valerian, 89
   Winnie the Pooh, 12
Sanicle (*Sanicula europaea*), 109
schizophrenia, 112
scrophula, 42
Scrophularia nodosa and *S. aquatica, see* Figwort
Scutellaria lateriflora and *S. galericulata, see* Skullcap
seeing the plants in a prescription, 94
Shaw, Non, xvii, xviii, xxviii
Shelf Fungus (*Ganoderma adspersum*), 27
Shen, 61
silibinin, 43 (f)
Silybum marianum syn. *Carduus marianus, see* Milk Thistle
Skullcap (*Scutellaria lateriflora, S. galericulata*), 13, **89**, 103
smudging
   Gorse (*Ulex europaeus*), 101
   Juniper (*Juniperus communis*), 58
   Sage (*Salvia officinalis*), 86
Sneezewort (*Achillea ptarmica*), 64
Solanum dulcamara, see Bittersweet
somatic tension, 11–12
Sonchus species, 66

soot sprites, 58 (f)
spleen, in traditional medicine, 19, 29, 38
splenic anger, 19
Spotted/Wild Geranium (*Geranium maculatum*), 56
St John's Wort (*Hypericum perforatum*), **87–89**
    facilitating lucid dreaming, 88
    folk tradition, 88
    for pain when near death, 87
    reaction to tea, 87
    and St John the Baptist, 88–89
storing sunsets, 109–110
storytelling, xviii, xix–xx, 107
Sulphur Polypore (*Laetiporus sulphureus*), 28
suppressed anger and the liver, 100–101
sweating herbs, 36
Symphytum officinale, see Comfrey
Symphytum tuberosum, see Tuberous Comfrey

tales, xix
Taraxacum officinale, see Dandelion
temperaments
    choleric humour, 3–8
    compared, 22
    and suitability of different geographies, 24
    melancholy humour, 18–21
    phlegmatic humour, 13–18
    and reaction to adversity, 23–24
    sanguine humour, 8–13
    two dominant humours, 22–23
thinking like plants, 111
Thistles, 21
Tilia species, see Lime Flowers
Thuja (*Thuja occidentalis*), 85
tradition versus direct plant knowledge, 96
traditional roots and phytochemical branches, 108–109
Treasure, Jonathan, xxi
Trifolium pratense, see Red Clover
trophorestorative, 50–51

Tuberous Comfrey (*Symphytum tuberosum*), 34
Turmeric (*Curcuma longa*), 13

ulcers, abscesses, boils, 9–10
unique understandings of herbs, 105
Urtica dioica, see Nettle

Valerian (*Valeriana officinalis*), 13, **89–90**
    in calming airy temperaments, 89
    caution in excitement-driven insomnia, 89–90
    as a French cavalry officer, 89
varicose ulcers, 11
vegetal philosophy, xxiii–xxiv, xxiii (f)
Vervain (*Verbena officinalis*), **90–91**
    a letting go herb, 90
    nauseant, 91
    reduces tension, 90
Viburnum opulus, see Cramp Bark
viral infections, 112–113
viriditas, xxii
vital spirits, 29, 37, 51–52, 61, 61 (f)
Vitex agnus-castus, see Chaste Berry

water, see phlegmatic humour
Water Betony, see Water Figwort
Water Figwort (*Scrophularia aquatica*), xxv, 41
weed medicine, 106
Weiss, Rudolph, xviii (f), 30, 53, 54
West, Cornel, xxi
Winston, David, 93–94
Woad (*Isatis tinctoria*), 29
womb, 64, 74, see Lady's Mantle, Mugwort, Raspberry Leaf
Wood Avens, see Herb Bennet
Wood Betony (*Betonica officinalis*), 82
Wormwood (*Artemisia absinthium*), **91**
writer's block, 19–20

Yarrow (*Achillea millefolium*), 47, 60, 71, 76, 113

Zanthoxylum americanum, Z. clava-herculis, see Prickly Ash